# Easeful Death

*Is There a Case for Assisted Dying?*

Mary Warnock
Elisabeth Macdonald

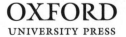

OXFORD
UNIVERSITY PRESS

# OXFORD

UNIVERSITY PRESS

Great Clarendon Street, Oxford OX2 6DP

Oxford University Press is a department of the University of Oxford.
It furthers the university's objective of excellence in research, scholarship,
and education by publishing worldwide in

Oxford  New York

Auckland  Cape Town  Dar es Salaam  Hong Kong  Karachi
Kuala Lumpur  Madrid  Melbourne  Mexico City  Nairobi
New Delhi  Shanghai  Taipei  Toronto

With offices in

Argentina  Austria  Brazil  Chile  Czech Republic  France  Greece
Guatemala  Hungary  Italy  Japan  Poland  Portugal  Singapore
South Korea  Switzerland  Thailand  Turkey  Ukraine  Vietnam

Oxford is a registered trademark of Oxford University Press
in the UK and in certain other countries

Published in the United States
by Oxford University Press Inc., New York

British Library Cataloguing in Publication Data

Data available

Library of Congress Cataloging-in-Publication Data

Warnock, Mary.
Easeful death : the case for assisted suicide? / Mary Warnock, Elisabeth Macdonald.
p.  ;  cm.
Includes bibliographical references and index.
ISBN-13: 978-0-19-953990-1 (alk. paper)  1. Euthanasia.  2. Assisted suicide.
3. Death–Social aspects.
[DNLM:  1. Euthanasia.  2. Suicide, Assisted.  3. Attitude to Death.  4. Ethics, Medical.
WB 60 W285e 2008]  I. Macdonald, Elisabeth.  II. Title.
R726.W36  2008
179.7-dc22                                        2007051134

Typeset by SPI Publisher Services, Pondicherry, India
Printed in Great Britain
on acid-free paper by
Clays Ltd, St Ives plc

ISBN  978-0-19-953990-1 (Hbk.)
ISBN  978-0-19-956184-1 (Pbk.)

1 3 5 7 9 10 8 6 4 2

# Contents

Darkling I listen; and, for many a time
I have been half in love with easeful death,
Called him soft names in many a mused rhyme,
To take into the air my quiet breath;
Now more than ever seems it rich to die,
To cease upon the midnight with no pain.

(John Keats, *Ode to a Nightingale* (1820), st. 6)

# Introduction

Why have we written this book now? The subject of assisted dying, voluntary euthanasia, and assisted suicide has long been widely debated; but there are good reasons for raising these thorny questions again at the present time.

In the British Parliament there have been three recent attempts, in 2003, 2004, and 2005, to legalize assisted death for those who requested it, and who were terminally ill. These attempts came through private members' bills, introduced into the House of Lords by Lord Joffe, an experienced and respected human rights lawyer. None of these Bills was proceeded with, the last being set aside in order that the issues might be examined by a Select Committee of the House, set up under the chairmanship of Lord Mackay of Clashfern, formerly Lord Chancellor. A fourth Bill was introduced in 2006 by Lord Joffe after the report of this Select Committee had been published and debated, but was not given a second reading and so lapsed.

All this parliamentary activity meant that the issues were kept in the public eye, not only in the UK but overseas. However, the scope of Lord Joffe's Bills was extremely limited, in that the right

## Introduction

to assisted dying was to be confined to those people who, being certified as of sound mind and unimpaired judgment, were terminally ill, that is, facing death within a matter of weeks or months, and who were suffering unbearable pain or distress. The fourth Bill sought to permit only assisted suicide, not euthanasia proper. That is, the Bill sought to legalize the action of a doctor who provided drugs that would enable the patient to kill himself, if he finally decided to do so, but the doctor would not be the killer (although provision was to be made so that where a patient was physically incapable of committing suicide, and satisfied the criteria set out in the Bill, a doctor might administer a lethal dose without fear of prosecution). This last Bill was debated, though not in detail, in May 2006. It is unlikely that there will be an immediate further attempt at legislation, in the UK at least, though it is certain that the issue will not go away, and a further attempt will be made in due course. Meanwhile, there is a legislative pause. It is therefore timely to collect the arguments together and examine them in a cool hour.

The question to be addressed is this: is it morally justifiable in some circumstances for a doctor or another person to end someone's life or help him to end it? And, if it is, is there a way of so changing the law that such an action may become not only morally but legally permitted? As the law stands, intentionally killing another person is murder, the most heinous offence of all, and the law prohibiting murder is often referred to as the cornerstone of the criminal law. Although suicide is no longer a crime in the UK (and never has been a crime in Scotland), assisting someone to commit suicide is a criminal offence, though the law is not implemented so as to visit the maximum sentence on someone found guilty of such an act.

There are various reasons why it has become a matter of urgency to try to find an answer to our question, even though it is by no means new. First, in an age when medical technology is constantly becoming more sophisticated, many people who die in hospital could be kept alive almost indefinitely on life support machines. For such people, death is not a matter of 'nature taking its course', but a matter of deliberate decision, not their own. There will come a time when someone, or some group of people, will decide not to resuscitate a patient if his heart fails, or will decide to give up all forms of treatment as 'futile' or unduly burdensome, and merely to keep him comfortable until he dies. The patient will have been allowed, if not helped, to die.[1]

Secondly, in the old days, an individual doctor, working alone or with the help of a district nurse, might decide on treatment or the withdrawal of treatment, relying on his own judgement, and pretty secure that his judgement would not be questioned either by the patient or the patient's relatives. The doctor's power was immense, and he was virtually unaccountable to anyone. Now, both because of the prevalence of hospital deaths, with the inevitable involvement of teams of doctors and nurses, and more generally because it is no longer regarded as proper for doctors to exercise such unquestioned decision-making powers, every decision has to be both transparent and justifiable. The question, not whether a patient will die, but when he shall be allowed to die, has to be capable of being openly discussed. And this, of course, leads to the question whether, when it is possible, the patient himself should not have a part, even a major part, in the discussion. In these changed circumstances it is highly desirable that society (all of whose members are potential patients, and all mortal) should think clearly about whether a patient should be legally entitled to decide to die. It is a question that affects us

## Introduction

all. It is not a clinical question, to be answered by the medical profession, but a social question for society at large.

Finally, we need urgently to consider practice in those few countries where some form of assisted death is already lawful. We need to see whether within these legislatures the consequences for society are turning out well or badly, whether there is reason to follow their lead or reject it. In the Netherlands, when a patient is deemed to be mentally competent to make the request and mean it, and when his suffering is agreed to be severe, he may lawfully be helped to die by his doctor, either by being helped to commit suicide or, more usually, by a lethal injection administered at home by his doctor. The patient does not have to be terminally ill before he can be so helped. Since 1973, Dutch doctors have been openly providing euthanasia on request, and if they were brought to court, they generally successfully pleaded necessity, to escape from a charge of murder. 'Necessity', which seems a rather strange mitigating plea in the circumstances, is a kind of 'force majeure', when the duty to preserve life, normally overriding, is itself outweighed by the duty to prevent suffering.[2]

This system understandably caused considerable uncertainty and anxiety among the medical profession, and in 2002 the law was changed by the introduction of the Termination of Life and Assisted Suicide (Review Procedures) Act, which regularized and legitimized the position of doctors. According to the terminology used in the Netherlands, 'euthanasia' means 'voluntary euthanasia' or 'voluntary assisted suicide'. So-called euthanasia, carried out supposedly in the best interests of the patient, but without his asking for it, is murder. (However there is some anecdotal evidence both that non-voluntary euthanasia is quite often carried out and that in hospital it is suggested to patients that they ask for euthanasia.) All cases where voluntary euthanasia has been carried out are supposed to be reported to the authorities; but the rate of reporting seems to be relatively low (just over 50 per cent), though this figure is naturally not easy to establish.

In Belgium, an Act of Parliament was also introduced in 2002, legalizing voluntary euthanasia but not assisted suicide. To qualify for euthanasia, the patient must 'be in a futile medical condition of constant physical or mental suffering that cannot be alleviated'. Again, cases of euthanasia are meant to be reported.

In the American State of Oregon, only assisted suicide is lawful, and that only for the terminally ill. The Death with Dignity Act was first passed as a result of individual initiative in 1994. However, it was passed then by only a small majority of the state electorate, and its implementation was halted by an injunction until it was put to the vote again and passed into state law by an increased majority in 1997. (That there was a certain element of defiance in the face of pressure from Federal Government cannot be doubted.) The evidence suggests that far more people ask to be given drugs that they could use if they found their condition becoming intolerable than actually use the drugs to end their lives. There is comfort simply in having a viable option to fall back on. Lord Joffe's last Bill, the Assisted Dying for the Terminally Ill Bill, 2006, was closely modelled on the law in Oregon, where he was impressed by the way it was working when he visited with other members of the House of Lords Select Committee.

Finally, in Switzerland, there are two relevant articles in the Penal Code. Article 114 makes voluntary euthanasia illegal; but Article 115 makes it lawful to help someone commit suicide if, and only if, the motive is 'entirely honourable', for example, to bring suffering to an end. Acting under this exemption, there have grown up several

## Introduction

voluntary organizations by joining which, for a fee, a patient may be helped to commit suicide at the time of his choice. The law does not actually require that the patient be assisted only if he is terminally ill; but this is laid down in a code of practice for the medical profession. One of the organizations, Dignitas, caters especially for overseas patients, who cannot get help in their own country. An increasing number of UK citizens are availing themselves of this service. But of course it is expensive, and stressful; and it means that people die sooner than they really want to, for fear that if they leave it too long they will become too ill to travel. To those who believe that there should be a general legal right to assisted dying, it is an outrage that those who can afford it are forced to go abroad for what they are, as they think, wrongfully denied in the UK, while most people cannot afford to avail themselves of this help.

It is against this background of different legislatures that the debate takes place in the UK, the USA, Australia, and elsewhere in the world. However, we believe that it is necessary to exercise caution in using other legislatures as a guide to how we should legislate in the UK. Those countries or states that have liberalized their laws have done so for different reasons and may have argued sometimes from the standpoint of rights, sometimes from that of compassion. Moreover, cultural differences between countries make it hard to generalize about the possible consequences of liberalization. Yet because the debate is so widespread and diverse, it is a good time to review the arguments for and against euthanasia.

The Report of the House of Lords Select Committee set up to consider Lord Joffe's penultimate Bill and the transcript of the oral evidence presented to the committee are immensely helpful in demonstrating the way people think and what they value in this complicated and emotionally laden field,[3] as are the Hansard reports of the House of Lords debates. We will refer to these sources frequently. Nevertheless, in what follows we do not confine ourselves to the narrow boundaries of Lord Joffe's Bills. For instance, his last Bill, following the example of the Oregon Death with Dignity Act (1994) was confined, as has been noted, to the legalization of assisted suicide. There is no doubt that the medical and nursing professions, hostile as many of them are to any form of assisted death, would nevertheless prefer the legalization of assisted suicide to that of euthanasia. We see no difference of principle between the two. Whether a doctor actually administers the lethal dose by injection or places a lethal dose by his patient's bed, with instructions to take it orally, what is at stake is whether he should be able, within the law, deliberately to bring about the death of his patient in response to a serious request from the patient that he do so, and when the wish to die is rational, fixed, and immovable.

Again, the Joffe Bill sought to legalize assisted suicide only for the terminally ill. Many people have raised objections to the Bill based on the ambiguity of the phrase 'terminally ill'; for, they say, though most people understand more or less what is meant by 'terminal illness' it is not capable of a definition precise enough for the purposes of the law. However, if at the heart of the debate is the rightness or wrongness of helping someone to die who can see no value to himself and no pleasure in his future life, the principle involved seems to be the same whether that life is to be long or short. Indeed, when someone has a progressive illness for which there is no cure, the length of time over which he will deteriorate may be one of the features of his case that most makes him want to die. And if his illness is not progressive, but renders him entirely helpless and dependent, it may be the length and unchanging tedium of the future that makes him sure that death is to be preferred to such a life.

**Introduction**

Lastly, Lord Joffe's Bill was to cover only those people who were mentally competent, and who have formally asked to die. Many of those whose objections to the Bill will be considered in due course use as their main argument that such voluntary euthanasia as was envisaged would lead 'inevitably' to a very different kind of euthanasia, the non-voluntary. Non-voluntary euthanasia is a concept at first sight so repugnant that it is difficult even to consider it rationally. Yet it occurs. Those in a permanent vegetative state may be deliberately caused to die; infants may be allowed to die if it is deemed to be in their best interests; and there is the suspicion that the mentally incompetent who are in hospital may be allowed or even helped to die. Even in the Netherlands, and certainly in other countries, including the UK, it is generally believed that in some cases doctors bring about the death of their patients in consideration of their best interest, when they have not asked that this should happen, but when their sufferings seem unbearable and further treatment futile. Doctors have to make such decisions frequently and, understandably, it is difficult, if not impossible, to know how often. We need to face the issue of justifiable euthanasia in whatever form it presents itself.

As we have said, the problem of euthanasia is a social, not a medical problem The issues are issues for us all. As the Select Committee Report put it: 'While opinion has often been divided within our committee...there has been unanimity on one point at least, that, while the most careful account must be taken of expert evidence, at the end of the day the acceptability of assisted suicide or voluntary euthanasia is an issue for society to decide.'[4]

Nobody can doubt that it is a moral problem. In some of the cases that we shall examine in the following chapters it may seem plainly morally right that a patient be helped to die. The central difficulty is to devise a law that would permit euthanasia in such cases and rule out other cases that would be morally dubious or abhorrent. Lord Joffe struggled to define in detail the circumstances of legitimate euthanasia, and include such safeguards as would make it impregnable to abuse. It may be that there is little possibility of successfully drafting such a Bill. Difficult though it may be legislation has been successfully drafted abroad. What, in a particular case, constitutes a strong moral imperative, namely to relieve someone's suffering when it has become too great, may be extremely difficult to generalize so as to determine a public policy. The moral imperative will come from an essentially personal motive, namely compassion, aroused by sympathy, our engagement with others, and the particular circumstances of the case; but when a Bill is drafted, it is the general, not the particular, with which the legislator must be concerned. He must ask what will be the consequences, for society as a whole, if this law reaches the statute book. It is the difference between private morality and public policy that may form the stumbling-block in the path of anyone seeking to change the law on euthanasia. We hope that a solution may be found. For, after all, private morality and public policy are not unconnected. Good laws cannot exist unless their foundation is in morality. What is needed is more open discussion to separate all the different considerations involved. To engender and, if possible, assist such a debate is the purpose of this book.

# 1 Fundamental Principles: The Nature of the Dispute

The issue before us is whether or not, for those who truly want it, assisted death should be a lawful option. Should they have a right to die at someone else's hand, or with someone else's active cooperation? If not, if there can be no circumstances in which it might be a duty deliberately to take the life of someone who, being perfectly sane and rational, is begging for death, then the argument is not contingent upon what might happen if the law were changed, but is absolute and a priori, independent of any particular facts. It is, in effect, the argument that human life is 'sacred'. If, on the other hand, there are circumstances in which it seems morally right to help to end the life of someone who wants to die, then the question is whether the law could be so changed as to make this not only morally right, but legally permissible.

It is often suggested that the two sides of this debate represent two conflicting principles: the principle of the sanctity of human life and the principle of autonomy. Indeed the House of Lords Select Committee, in composing their report, structured it so as to turn on the conflict between these two principles. We return to a more detailed analysis of what is meant by the sanctity of human life in

## Fundamental Principles

Chapter 6, and will there consider the role of religion in the whole debate, while recognizing that it is not only the religious who claim to be guided by the principle. For the time being, the principle may be taken to assert that it must always be better for someone to be alive than dead, and that the argument against deliberately killing must always trump all other arguments. We turn now, therefore, to the principle of autonomy. This principle is generally supposed to be that upon which those who advocate a change in the law chiefly base their case.

The principle of patient autonomy has become one of the fundamental principles that are taught to medical students in their compulsory ethics courses. The principle was first set out as one of four that lay at the root of medical ethics by Beauchamp and Childress in a book that has become a kind of sacred text.[1] The four principles are those of *beneficence* (the doctor must be well-intentioned towards his patient and aim to do good); *non-maleficence* (the doctor must avoid harming his patient); *autonomy* (the doctor must treat his patient as a rational human being capable of making choices and possessed of free will); and *justice* (the doctor must distribute resources, including time and skill, fairly between his patients). The authors never pretended that these principles might not sometimes be in conflict with each other. For example, it is obvious that the principle of autonomy might conflict with that of justice, if what one patient wanted could be supplied only at the expense of others; or with that of beneficence, if a doctor believed that what the patient chose would not be in his best interest. All they argued was that each of them must be at least considered, in cases where a doctor found himself asking what, morally, he ought to do. Our concern is only with the principle of autonomy.

The principle is often said to be derived from the moral philosophy of Immanuel Kant; and there is a kinship between them. Kant's aim was to demonstrate how it was possible, in a world newly shown by Newton to be governed entirely by the laws of physics, for human beings yet to be free moral agents. He argued that, in all respects except one, human beings were part of the natural world and subject, like all of nature, to physical laws. The one unique feature of a human being was his possession of reason, and this could be identified with his free will. The only thing in the world that could be good in the specifically moral sense was the human will; and this will enabled human beings, alone of animals, to give themselves rational and absolute laws, imperatives, which must be obeyed on pain of contradiction, even if obedience to them went against their desires. These laws, like Newton's, apply universally, though each must discover them for himself, through his own reason. Thus, for example, in a situation of scarcity, such as a drought, where a rationing of water is imposed, it is morally wrong to take more than one's share, because reason dictates that one cannot will this to be the universal law. If everyone obeyed the instinct to make an exception for himself, then all would die of thirst. Kant believed that it was the irrationality of willing that one should take more than one's share that made it imperative not to do so. Just as one cannot not accept the logical truth that, if $a$ is greater than $b$ and $b$ is greater than $c$, then $a$ is greater than $c$, so one must accept the force of the argument against universally making exceptions to the rationing of water. The difference is that in the latter case the reasoning is practical, affecting not just our thoughts but our actions. So one formulation of the moral, categorical, imperative is 'Never act on a principle that could not be conceived as a universal principle'. Now, since every human being has this same power to act as a rational moral agent, and it is the possession of the power to make moral choices that makes him human, it would be impossible to act on a universal principle that would deny this power to another human being. The moral or rational law requires that people should be treated as free, choice-making creatures, as one is oneself. So another formulation of the categorical imperative is that one must never treat another human being as a mere means to an end, but always as an end in himself. We must not make his choices for him; they must spring from his own autonomous will. This, after all, is what 'autonomy' means: making one's own laws, adopting one's own principles. From these formulations of the categorical imperative our duty can be deduced; and a morally meritorious action is one performed as a duty.

So the morally good doctor must not only avoid using his patient for his own ends (to prove a theory, say, or to advance clinical research) but he must allow him to exercise his own will, as a fellow human being. And here we have the medical principle of autonomy. There is no doubt that this principle harmonizes with the modern distrust of medical paternalism, and with the egalitarianism that puts doctors and their patients (or 'service users' as we are now taught to call them) on an equal footing. It also accounts for the general insistence on informed consent. On the other hand, Kant's moral theory was nothing if not grand. Absolutist and derived from his whole enormous critical philosophy, he was prepared to accept the paradoxes it threw up (for example, that actions undertaken from motives other than pure reason or the demands of duty, from pity, for instance, or love, can have no moral worth). The consistency of his whole critique was paramount. And even the greatest enthusiast for the primacy of patient autonomy among the principles of good medical practice must admit that there are legitimate limits to patient choice. A patient, even a rich, paying patient, cannot force a doctor to give him the treatment of his choice, if in the doctor's judgement it would be futile. The patient's preferences cannot always outweigh the doctor's superior knowledge and professional expertise. The difficulty lies in determining where precisely these limits should be drawn; and so we are back where we started. Granted that a patient should be allowed some say in his treatment, and should not be treated against his will, should his autonomy extend to choosing his time and manner of death? May a patient choose to die?

It may seem more plausible to derive the principle of autonomy from the idea of patients' rights than from any philosophical theory of individual autonomy. And this is certainly the language that would be preferred in the twenty-first century. But this, in fact, gets us no further. If we ask, 'Has a patient a right to choose to die?', the answer either depends on the state of the law, in which case in the UK and most of Europe and America the answer is an unequivocal 'No', or it depends on whether or not we think that to choose to die is a natural or human right, regardless of what legal rights a person may have under any particular legislature. But there is no definitive list of human rights. Each disputed case must be settled in court.

In the UK in the year 2002 there was an important case that was widely debated. This was the case of Diane Pretty. Mrs Pretty suffered from motor neurone disease, a progressive and incurable illness, which leads first to weakness and then to paralysis of all the limbs. Mental function is not usually impaired, but in the last stages of the disease the patient is totally dependent on others. Diane Pretty did not want to reach the stage when she would have increasing difficulty in speaking, swallowing, and breathing. She was incapable of herself performing any act of suicide, and she did not want her GP to assist her, since for him to do so would have been an unlawful act that would damage him professionally. She therefore requested that her husband should assist her, and sought an assurance from the Director of Public Prosecutions that if he did so he would not be prosecuted. The DPP refused to give her this assurance, and so she took her request to court. Her request for assistance to die was refused by two courts in the UK, and she finally appeared before the European Court of Human Rights in Strasburg, where her request was again refused. The judgment was that, though she had a right to life, she had no right to death. This response was no more than a tautology, in that what she was asking was that she should be granted the right (or be told that she already possessed it under a higher legislature) that she had repeatedly been told she did not possess under British legislation. However, the European Court deemed that the British courts had relied on a constitutional law that it would not seek to overturn. The judges found that none of her Convention rights were infringed by the terms of the Suicide Act 1961, under which it is a criminal offence to assist another to commit suicide; and member states of the EU are permitted to legislate according to the morals of their own community. So the fact that elsewhere in Europe she could lawfully have sought help to die was not relevant to the position of legislators in the UK. In simpler terms, the European Court endorsed the moral judgment of the British courts. It could be argued that, since suicide is a lawful option for those capable of committing it, to refuse the option of suicide to a disabled person is discrimination, which is unlawful both in European and UK law. But perhaps assisting someone to kill himself cannot count as a 'service' of which the disabled must not be deprived. At any rate, this line of reasoning was not pursued in the court.[2]

This case, which was part of the background to Lord Joffe's Bills, attracted enormous sympathy for the patient and others in her position. And it is clear that, although the question of rights was settled against her, the moral question remained open to dispute. Ought she to have been granted a right to die? Should everyone have such a right, to exercise if they choose? If she had been able, she would have committed suicide, and suicide is no longer a crime. If she had been subject to intrusive and distressing treatment, such as chemotherapy, she could have chosen to forgo any further treatment, and thus caused her own death. This is the legal right of any patient, even if medical opinion regards the choice as ill-judged. (Since no treatment may be carried out without a patient's consent, a doctor who persisted in treating a patient against her will would be guilty of assault.) But Mrs. Pretty fell into neither of these categories, so all she could do was wait for her inevitable and dreaded death, which came just as she feared it would. She certainly exercised no autonomy in the manner of her death.

But the question may be raised whether Diane Pretty and her supporters who thought she should be helped to die were entirely relying on the principle of autonomy in putting forward their case. They may have been. She herself was plainly a woman of principle, and thought it wrong in principle that her husband or her GP should suffer punishment on her behalf; and she may genuinely have wanted, above all, that other people in her predicament should have the acknowledged right to be helped to die. If this was her motive, then it would be true to say that her claim to assisted suicide was based on the principle of autonomy.

In many cases, however, though this principle may be part of the motive for requesting help to die, another part of it is more personal. It is simply that a patient finds that he cannot any longer bear his increasing dependence and helplessness. There are many people who suffer acutely before the foreseen end of their life, and who ask that they be helped to die not on account of any principle but on account of the very nature of their suffering, what they see as the total indignity of being unable to do anything for themselves or have any control over the way their life is lived. They hate the enforced intimacy of severe illness. They were once, like the heroic human beings envisaged in Kant's moral theory, people of free will, choosing what they did and independently deciding how they should live. Now that that has gone, their life has no value for them. They could doubtless bear the pain, if there were any hope of regaining control of their lives. They hanker for autonomy, not so much as a matter of principle, applicable to everyone, but because they personally intensely prefer freedom to the slavery to illness in which they find themselves. In her speech in support of Lord Joffe's Bill, Baroness Murphy, a specialist in geriatric psychiatry, described these people thus:

These people are quite distinctive personalities and often not very easy patients. They hate above all the prospect of total dependence on others, detest losing control and are unwilling to sacrifice their individuality to institutional norms. They want to be in charge of their fate, and it is the uncertainty about the end that is distressing to an unbearable degree…What causes their unbearable suffering is not remediable by medicine nor psychological supports but by respecting their wishes and supporting them to choose their own time of death.[3]

The House of Lords Select Committee acknowledged that this was so. They recognized the existence of some patients, perhaps a minority, for whom palliative care, however skilful, would never be wholly successful, and whose wish to end their lives was overwhelming. Many of these patients, even if not actually paralysed, would find it impossible to commit suicide, being under constant surveillance in hospital or hospice, with no chance even to accumulate drugs with which to end their lives. In the evidence to the Select Committee, Dr Carole Dacombe, medical director of St Peter's Hospice in Bristol and an experienced practitioner in palliative care, described these people:

They often are people who have a long life history of seeking control over their own destiny, of wishing to plan their lives for themselves. They often are people who, despite having explored various faith structures or spiritual concepts that some of us find are a great help and support to us in life have either rejected them or failed to find in them sufficient solace to see them through the final stages of whatever illness it is that they are dealing with....If I truly believe in the principles by which we work in palliative care, which are to respect our patients, to respect their need for respect, for dignity and choice, I need to be prepared to listen to patients who wish to request [assistance to die].[4]

The Select Committee referred to this horror at loss of dignity and control as 'existential autonomy', that is, autonomy not as a right to be defended but as an experienced condition, and one which alone gave value to life. For people such as those described by Baroness Murphy and Dr Dacombe, autonomy, far from standing in opposition to the sanctity of life, is actually what makes a life 'sacred', at least for the person who lives it.

It is for this reason that we do not believe it is adequate to identify the dispute between those who oppose assisted dying and those who defend it with a clash between the principle of the sanctity of life and that of autonomy. Most people are not entirely Kantian in their concept of morality. They do not hold that all moral choices are matters of principle, or categorical imperatives that must have universal application and that arise from reason alone. On the contrary, they hold that morally good actions may often be motivated by what in the eighteenth century used to be called 'moral sentiment'. Good people do good things because, in Jane Austen's words, they 'feel as they ought'. And these moral sentiments are such as themselves to give rise to imperatives. If we find an animal caught in a trap, alive but in terrible pain, we feel that we cannot leave it, we must release it or kill it, to end its agony. This is an imperative that arises from sympathy (we understand pain, even the pain of foxes) and compassion. Thus we are compelled to believe that many people who would have supported Diane Pretty's plea to the Court of Human Rights would have done so out of compassion and sympathy, not out of principle. They could not bear to contemplate her suffering.

Compassion is not a principle. And this is precisely where the trouble lies when we try to change the law. If morality, as Kant supposed, were really a matter only of imperatives derived from universal principles, then there should be no conflict between morality and the law. Both the principles by which we should live, our duty, and the laws themselves would apply to everyone in society, as the hosepipe ban in times of drought applies to everyone in the area, and that includes me; and there can be no moral justification for my making an exception for myself, however tempted I may be to do so. But compassion, despair, pity, and sympathy are sentiments that are not susceptible to such generalizations. They arise, and dictate to us, in specific situations. Together, they could be said to constitute an important part of my conscience, my sense of what I owe to other people. In a completely different context, that of homosexual couples adopting children, the archbishop of Canterbury is reported as saying that the law must never inhibit conscience;[5] but the trouble is that it sometimes does. If what the law forbids and what I feel I must do are in conflict then if I follow my conscience I must risk paying the penalty. And this is exactly the case in the UK with regard to so-called mercy killing. In one sense, I must do what I think right, whatever the law. But the law and morality are not totally separate. I am inhibited in doing what the law forbids, not only because I may fear the consequences, but also because in a democracy the law is the voice of an elected parliament looking towards a common good, a commonality in which I share. Under a tyrannical government, where democratic principles have been abandoned, the attitude of morally good people towards the law would radically change. This fact lies at the heart of the need we feel at the present time to consider, as a matter of urgency, whether the law with regard to 'mercy killing' should not perhaps be changed. Hard cases may make bad law; but if there are too many hard cases, if there are too many cases where people's compassionate conscience dictates what the law forbids, then it must be made a question whether the law is wrong. The difficulty is to incorporate compassion into the law.

In the evidence to the Select Committee the Revd Professor Robin Gill, representing the archbishop of Canterbury and the House of Bishops, made manifest, albeit in somewhat bumbling style, the nature of the difficulty, where we believe the centre of the true dispute resides:

As some of you know, I made a submission myself for Diane Pretty. I did it entirely on compassionate grounds. I thought that her case represented a very very strong case indeed for voluntary euthanasia and if it was simply a matter of her and no one else and not other people, I believe that this was as strong a case as you get and on compassionate grounds one should certainly reach out for it. When I made my submission I also made it clear that ... [t]he issue of legalising voluntary euthanasia is not simply a religious versus non-religious issue, there are divisions on both sides, but that for my part I was not convinced on compassionate grounds. In the end I concluded, as my Church has concluded, that more people, more vulnerable people will be made more vulnerable if we change the law in favour of legalising euthanasia.[6]

We can hear, in these words, the conflict between compassion, moral sentiment, and the rule of law or respect for the common as opposed to the individual good. (And it is noticeable that, even when finally coming down on the side of the law and against his earlier submission, Professor Gill does not invoke the a priori principle of the sanctity of life, but the apparently empirical argument that a change in law would, in practice, do more harm than good.)

And so the question posed by this book is this: can we devise a law that allows us to relieve the suffering of those who want to die, without endangering others who do not want to? Can we reconcile what may be an intensely experienced private imperative, arising from compassion or love, with a public policy for the common good? It is to be hoped that the following chapters may throw light on this problem, though they will not solve it.

In December 2006, the Law Commission published a report, entitled *Murder, Manslaughter and Infanticide*. The seventh chapter of the report considers the question whether so-called mercy killing should be a separate crime, attracting a lesser penalty than homicide. In paragraph 7.29 the commissioners write:

There remains the possibility of a tailor-made offence or partial defence which is centred on the concept of 'acting out of compassion'. However we continue to believe that there would need to be a much wider debate before concluding that the concept of 'compassion' as a motive is in itself a suffi-ciently secure foundation for a 'mercy killing' offence or partial defence.[7]

It is to this debate that we hope to contribute.

However, before entering into the details of the debate, there is one argument against a change in the law of murder that needs to be noticed, and, in our view, set aside. This is the argument put for-ward with passion by those medical practitioners, both doctors and nurses, who specialize in palliative care for the dying. They contend that, if physician-assisted suicide or euthanasia were to become a lawful option, palliative care would suffer. Resources would be with-drawn and research into pain control would cease to attract funding. At the present time, in the UK and elsewhere in the world, what is needed is more not less palliative care, more not fewer resources directed towards it. There have been great advances in the science of pain management, but more research is needed. And above all, at present far too few patients have access to good, specialist palliative care. The hospice movement, started as a private charity and still largely supported by charitable gifts, is directed almost exclusively to cancer patients at the end of their lives. Though the character of the movement is changing, it is not, and cannot be, adequate to the needs of an ageing population, nor to the needs of people, of whatever age, suffering from other incurable and often unbearable conditions such as AIDS or motor neurone disease. Any legislation that stood in the way of the needed increase and wider spread of palliative care should be opposed.

We entirely agree with the proposition that palliative care should be far more widely available, and its increased availability and improvement should be among the top priorities of medical policy. But, in our view, there will always be those, perhaps few, for whom palliative care is not the solution to their suffering. There are those, as we have already suggested, who quite genuinely would prefer death, and who long to die sooner rather than later. The premise upon which the argument for palliative care rather than physician-assisted death rests is that it is always better to live than die, even if one passionately wants to die. And there are those, whose plight we also consider in the following chapters, who are living on for an indefinite time with no prospect of recovery, who are either unconscious, or who cannot face the futility of the life that lies ahead of them. For these people the question must arise whether a change in the law cannot be devised to let them die.

In any case, it is not necessarily true that palliative care would suffer if physician-assisted death were to become lawful in certain specified circumstances. Research into palliative care might become more intensive, when the alternative was that a patient might request his own death. Fewer people would need to do so, as palliative care improved and became more widely available.

# 2 Types of Euthanasia

So far, we have spoken of assisted death, and made little distinction between the forms that assisted death may take. The following three chapters will be concerned with the problems that have arisen in different kinds of cases, and what has been their outcome.

The first distinction to be drawn is between assisted death that has been asked for by a patient, and that which has not. This chapter and the next will be concerned with requested death. The paradigm case of physician-assisted dying is that of a patient who is at the end of his life, who knows that he is dying of some incurable disease, and who asks his doctor that he be helped to die before his suffering becomes more intense.

It is plain that, if such assisted death were to be permitted by law, the patient's request would have somehow to be formalized, written and signed before witnesses, or, if writing was impossible, at least uttered before witnesses like an oath. Many people when their suffering was especially bad might say that they wished they were dead; but this would not be enough to ensure that they really had a fixed intent to die, that they would commit suicide if they could, and would not change their mind. Such formalization would be incorporated in any new legislation, as it was in Lord Joffe's Bills.

The case of Diane Pretty has already been described. But it must be noticed in this context that it is not only the paralysed who cannot commit suicide without assistance. For people who are ignorant of medicine, it is very difficult to guess what dosage of any particular drug would be lethal; and in any case for those who are in hospital or a hospice, it is impossible to build up a private store even of those pills that have been prescribed. Medication is brought round in the prescribed quantity at the appropriate time, and any pills not swallowed are removed. There is, furthermore, a considerable risk that even a seriously attempted suicide may fail, and this may lead to intensified suffering. In the Netherlands, where both assisted suicide and euthanasia are permitted, when a patient chooses assisted suicide, it is part of the duty of a doctor to look after the patient, and if necessary actively assist him to die if his attempted suicide fails. Euthanasia must take over, where suicide has failed.

Indeed, it is not always easy to sustain a distinction between assisted suicide and voluntary euthanasia. For, in the case of Diane Pretty and others in her condition, someone would have had either to administer a lethal dose, or to give her a lethal injection. She could do nothing for herself. Presumably in the State of Oregon, where only assisted suicide is permitted, her request for help to die would have been turned down.

Lord Joffe's last Bill, whose progress through Parliament was aborted in May 2006, was, he said, modelled on the Death with Dignity Act that had been in force in Oregon for eight years. Yet it was entitled 'Assisted Dying for the Terminally Ill', not 'Assisted Suicide' precisely because it contained an attempt to provide for those who could not actually kill themselves, because they could not swallow, even if the necessary medication was provided. However the relevant clause in the Bill is not without ambiguity. It is clause 1(a)(ii), which entitles a doctor to assist a patient to die not merely by prescribing medication but 'in the case of a patient for whom it is impossible or inappropriate orally to ingest that medication, by prescribing and providing such means of self-administration of that medication as will enable the patient to end his own life'. But Diane Pretty would not have been able to put the lethal drug into a feeding tube when she had to be fed by intubation. However, this first clause also allows that someone else may lawfully work in conjunction with the physician to bring about the desired result. This, as some opponents of the Bill were quick to point out, comes 'to the very brink of euthanasia'. For if her husband or a sympathetic nurse had put the medication into the feeding tube at her request, under the proposals of this clause, had the Bill been enacted, it would presumably have been a lawful act, and it would have been difficult to argue that it was not an act of euthanasia. Doubtless if Joffe's Bill had proceeded to a committee stage, this issue would have been clarified. But, given the intention to help patients such as Diane Pretty, it is plausible to argue that no distinction in principle was made in the Bill between assisted suicide and euthanasia. The fact of the matter is that euthanasia is what Diane Pretty would have to have had, if she were to have assisted death at all. Of course Lord Joffe could not use the word 'euthanasia' in the title of the Bill. That word produces a knee-jerk reaction of horror, which is hardly lessened even if one is careful to speak always of 'voluntary euthanasia'. Whatever the realities, in the UK at least, it seems that no Bill with the word in its title would have much chance of finding its way onto the statute book at the present time.

## Types of Euthanasia

In any case, though prefacing 'euthanasia' with 'voluntary' rules out killing people who do not want to be killed, it also rules out killing people who are incapable of either wanting or not wanting to die, when, for instance, they are in a permanent vegetative state. And, as we shall see, the moral questions about deliberately ending life arise acutely in just such cases (see Chapter 5). Nor does the word 'voluntary' do justice to the passionate wish to die that is the characteristic of the people whom Lord Joffe's Bill sought to help. These people are not just 'willing' or 'consenting' to die; they are begging to be allowed to die; 'willing themselves' to die, perhaps, but this rather childish usage is not what 'voluntary' means. In fact, the word 'voluntary' ought perhaps to be dropped from the discussion. We should instead speak of 'asked for' or 'requested' or 'chosen' death, cumbersome though this may be, and contrast this with a death that is deliberately brought about but without the patient's request.

Diane Pretty's case is not unique. Another example is that of a Canadian woman, Sue Rodriguez, who suffered from amyotrophic lateral sclerosis. Her condition was progressive and incurable, but her likely survival time could not be calculated with certainty. She had young children, and wanted to live as long as possible because of them, and therefore did not wish to commit suicide immediately, although at this stage she could probably still have managed it. Instead, she petitioned the Canadian Supreme Court for help to die at that time in the future when her life would be intolerable, and she would be unable to kill herself without help. Her appeal was made under the Canadian Charter of Rights and Freedoms, but it was turned down by a narrow margin.[1] In the end Mrs Rodriguez did get help to commit suicide when she could no longer tolerate her life, but only through the good offices of a doctor friend who was willing to risk a criminal charge, and who administered a lethal injection.

Considering these two cases, we may conclude that it is not helpful to try to make a legal distinction between assisted suicide and euthanasia. Moreover, it is not helpful, or fair, to distinguish terminal from progressive illness as a justification for assisted dying. Certainly Sue Rodriguez was not terminally ill when she first appealed to the court; and it could probably be argued that Diane Pretty was not either. Someone who would be agreed to be terminally ill is someone already in the last stages of the disease that is killing him. He is certain not only that he is dying but that he has only a few weeks, or even days, to live. The argument in favour of helping only those who are terminally ill to die if they so wish is partly based on the thought that this is simply 'easing the passing', that there is so little life left to them that it cannot matter if they are allowed to forgo this short span. But the fact that the length of his potential life is short does not seem relevant to the question whether or not it can ever be lawful to grant a person's request for death.

Indeed, the reason for his request for death may be precisely because his life will probably be long. It is what his life is like that counts: its quality, as he perceives it. In the Netherlands there is no restriction of lawful euthanasia to the terminally ill. The basis for acceding to a request is 'hopeless and unbearable suffering', and has nothing to do with life expectancy.[2]

And this brings us to another kind of case, a kind that would not in any interpretation fall under a law permitting assisted death for the terminally ill. This kind of case may be exemplified by that of a Canadian woman, Nancy B., which ended in a definite and general ruling by a Quebec judge, Mr Justice Dufour, that 'people have the right to demand that life support be removed, even when they are not dying, if they find life intolerable in the circumstances in which they must live it'.[3] Nancy B. was 25 years old and suffering from a rare neurological condition, Guillain-Barre syndrome, for which there was no cure. She was paralysed from the neck down. She said of herself: 'The only thing I have is television and looking at the walls. It's enough. It's been two and a half years that I've been on this thing and I think I've done my share.' Her doctor had said that she might go on living on the respirator for many years; but the respirator was turned off after the judge's ruling and she died soon after. This was in 1992.

A similar later case, that of an English woman, known only as Ms B, is discussed in more detail in Chapter 8, where it is used to illustrate the extreme difficulty that the medical professions experience with the thought that they should deliberately bring the life of a patient to an end.[4]

Whether Nancy B. should be described as having been helped to commit suicide or having been granted asked-for euthanasia seems a trivial matter compared with the fact that the judge decided that, in her case and, he implied, that of others like her, she had a right to die.

There is one other kind of requested death that must be considered, but because it raises some unique and uniquely intractable problems, it will form the subject of a separate chapter, Chapter 3.

# 3  Psychiatric Assisted Suicide

I n this chapter we consider a class of cases not very often mentioned in the context of euthanasia, namely requests for assisted death from those who suffer severe and recurrent mental illness. Such cases may present acute moral dilemmas for doctors and carers who have responsibility for the mentally ill. We hold that the problems raised should be acknowledged. But we do not believe that any solution to them is likely until there is greater clarity about the nature of mental illness, and about the suffering that some psychiatric patients may endure.

In his oral evidence to the House of Lords Select Committee, Dr Legemaate, chief legal counsel to the Royal Dutch Medical Society, replying to a question from the chairman, Lord Mackay of Clashfern, stated that the basis for euthanasia in the Netherlands is the 'unbearable and hopeless suffering' of the patient.[1] Dr Legemaate agreed that most of those who were assisted to die were terminally ill, and many of them were old; but he went on to say 'we do not exclude the rather exceptional situations in which, for instance, somebody who is 55 and has a very severe but incurable mental illness which relates to a situation of hopeless and unbearable suffering asks for suicide. We have had these cases now and then. Not many. But they are not excluded.' Thus both parts of the dual criterion for the legality of euthanasia in the Netherlands may be satisfied by such a person: first, that the doctor confirms that his suffering is hopeless and unbearable, and secondly that he has seriously and responsibly requested that he be helped to die. It is clear from this response that suffering from severe mental illness is not taken necessarily to render a patient incompetent, nor to entail that his request be set aside. Nor is 'unbearable suffering' confined to physical pain. There has been one case in the UK in which these presumptions appear to be shared. In 1994 a man, C, was under mental health care and had been diagnosed as suffering from paranoid schizophrenia. An English court upheld his right to refuse treatment, even though his doctors believed that it would save his life. Moreover the court held that if C should later lapse into incompetence his decision should remain binding.[2]

Yet such cases are fraught with difficulty and are likely to produce initial outrage. Most lay people, at least, would probably argue that suicide or a determination to die usually arises out of depression, which is a mental illness, and which may call into question the competence of the sufferer to make reasonable decisions. Moreover, depression is often capable of being alleviated by drugs, even if it is likely to recur. This optimism explains why people think it right to intervene if they can to prevent suicide, and this is at least part of the reason why assisted suicide is still a crime under the present law. To allow someone, let alone assist him, to kill himself is to squander a life which could be made more tolerable if help were to hand. People who are close to or who are responsible for someone who commits suicide are very likely to blame themselves bitterly for not foreseeing what was going to happen and for not intervening to get treatment for the victim, to prevent the terrible waste.

And so we tend immediately to think that psychiatrists, whose task it is to treat and alleviate mental illness have a particular duty to prevent their patients from committing suicide, and should never agree to their requests for help to do so, and indeed should do everything to restrain them. After all, suicide is not a mere symptom of depression, like being unable to get up in the morning or loss of appetite. It is not something that can be moderately or partially relieved. It is the final end, the worst thing of all. If a patient is killed by his doctor or offered a lethal dose to take by himself, then that doctor is, in effect, saying 'your suffering is worse than death, and death alone can relieve it'. And this is indeed the message that the patient has himself accepted.

On the other hand, and against the gut reaction we are all likely to experience when we first think about it, it may be argued that there are situations where suicide is a rational choice, though a sad one. In the case of Diane Pretty, for example, her desire to commit suicide was based on a perfectly rational preference for avoiding the inevitable and clearly foreseen horror of her death, if she allowed 'nature to take its course'. Suicide was in her best interest. Had she been physically able to take her own life she would have done so, nor are there many who would have failed to understand her choice. There would have been no grounds for saying that she killed herself only because she was suffering from a clinical depression which could be cured. There is no evidence to suggest that she was depressed. Considering such cases as hers, it must be wrong, and insulting, to argue that all suicide is the outcome of mental incompetence. Moreover it is not the case that all mental illness can be cured.

## Psychiatric Assisted Suicide

Diane Pretty's case clearly illustrates how much more at home we are with the concept of physical than of mental illness. If it were possible to show a defect or irreversible degeneration of the brain in every case of mental illness, then we might be able to deem some psychiatric patients to be rational in their desire to commit, or be helped to commit, suicide before things got worse for them. Their situation would be like that of Diane Pretty. But so far this is not possible. Even psychiatrists seem unable certainly to distinguish a mental illness that can be treated and one that cannot, to say nothing of a so-called personality disorder, for which therapy is inappropriate. There is still widespread confusion about what counts as a diagnosable mental illness. Some people, even those accustomed to distinguishing things that differ, still talk about a 'disease of the mind', as if the mind were an organ like the liver. The vocabulary, as well as the concept, of mental illness is confused.

So the question must be asked whether, where the mental illness is the cause of potential suicide, efforts must always be made to prevent it; or where a rational request has been made for assistance in dying that request must always be refused. Can a moral case be made out for permitting it? Should a doctor ever make it easier for a patient who has been profoundly depressed and fears a recurrence to commit suicide? Or offer help to a patient in the grip of a recurring mental illness, temporarily in remission, to do so?

A patient who is physically ill has the right to refuse treatment; and he may make an advance decision (see Chapter 5) to the effect that he now refuses treatment for his future self, should he become incompetent. We have seen that, in the case of C, a patient suffering from mental illness was unusually accorded the same right. Yet generally, a patient suffering with an acute but episodic mental illness is given no such right. In the Code of Practice on Advanced

Decisions published by the British Medical Association in 1995 (after the case of C) the authors say: 'Advance Statements appear to have only limited value in relation to the treatment of recurrent episodic mental illness. This is a unique area in which patients are unable to refuse compulsory detention and treatment for mental disorder authorized by mental health legislation, though notice of their preferred treatment may be helpful.' And in a judgment from the Court of Appeal,[3] Lord Phillips of Worth Matravers found that even if a patient, as a result of enforced treatment, became competent to take decisions, it still did not constitute an infringement of human rights if he were treated compulsorily, provided that the treatment could be shown to be a 'medical necessity'. The reason for society's reluctance to allow those suffering from mental illness to refuse treatment is of course the fear that they might cause harm to others if they are not 'sectioned', or compulsorily committed to hospital under the Mental Health Act. But the disparity between the respect for a physically sick patient's autonomy and that for the mentally sick is being increasingly questioned. Society seems to react quite differently to their sufferings.

The kind of suffering that may be experienced by someone in the grip of an episodic mental illness may be illustrated by the example of a well-known Washington figure, Philip Graham (though as it happened he did not have to seek help to kill himself). In her autobiography,[4] his widow Katharine Graham, long-time owner-president and publisher of the *Washington Post*, tells the terrible story of Philip's mental illness and final suicide. A charismatic, domineering, and immensely successful man who had succeeded Katharine's father at the *Post* and was her predecessor there, he began, while in office, to suffer acute depression. He consulted a psychiatrist, who belonged to the then fashionable school of psychiatry which, starting from French sociology, became well-known through the writings of such broadly anti-establishment figures as Thomas Szasz and R.D. Laing. These doctors repudiated the orthodox idea of mental illness and treatment by drugs, and were often unwilling to attach names to mental conditions as if they were analogous to physical diseases. In consequence it was a long time before Katharine realized that her husband was manic depressive. In his manic phase, he was capable of wild extravagance, as well as destructive rages and widespread human damage. During one such phase, he left Katharine and their four children, and went to live with a young Australian journalist on one of the many farms he had bought almost at random. But then his depression returned. He came home, having abandoned the journalist, and after two days went back to the nursing home where he had been treated before. He appeared to make good progress. But, Katharine wrote, 'worry about his actions and what he had done to himself, his life and to all of us was the main thing on his mind—that, plus the knowledge that not only had it happened, but it would happen again'. After a few weeks in the nursing home, he became passionately determined to come home for a weekend and to spend it with Katharine at their country farm. Opinion among his doctors was divided, but in the end he won them over to the view that a break would do him good. So he and Katharine were driven to the farmhouse, sat on the porch having lunch together and listening to music, and then went upstairs for a nap. After a few minutes he got up, saying that he was going to a different bedroom that he sometimes used, and there he shot himself with one of the many shotguns kept at the farm. Katharine wrote of how she blamed herself for letting him leave the bedroom on his own. She added:

It had never occurred to me that he must have planned the whole day at Glen Welby to get at his guns....I believe that Phil came to the sad conclusion that he would never again lead a normal life. I think he realized that the illness would recur. However he himself defined his illness, Phil was well aware of the damaging effects of it on others and on him. I think he felt he'd done such harm the last time around that he just couldn't deal with it. It was unendurable to him not only that he couldn't make any of it right, but that he might cause more hurt again.

For someone who had been such a dynamic decision-maker, it must have been totally intolerable to have lost control of his own life. Suicide would at least be his own decision and his own act. And it was rational to decide, at whatever cost, to avoid harming his family again.

The psychiatrists at the nursing home presumably reproached themselves for having allowed Graham to leave, and probably considered that, in some sense, in doing so they had condemned him to death, though they themselves played no active part in it. But it may be that, short of keeping him incarcerated against his will for the rest of his life, there was nothing that would have prevented his suicide sooner or later. He needed no help in order to kill himself. There were dozens of guns at his farm, he knew how to use them and was a man of resolution. But suppose that his circumstances had been different, and he had needed a lethal drug to carry out his purpose. Given that he was diagnosed as severely mentally ill, would it have been morally right for a doctor to help him? In the Netherlands it would have been a case of lawful euthanasia. In this country and most other countries it would be homicide; and even supplying drugs, knowing or strongly suspecting the patient's motive in asking for them, it would be assisting a suicide, a criminal, though lesser, offence.

## Psychiatric Assisted Suicide

But psychiatrists must often find themselves faced with a moral dilemma. And these dilemmas stem from the degree to which doctors should allow their patients a part in determining their own treatment. Two other cases may be considered, both of which were discussed in an issue of the periodical *Philosophy, Psychiatry and Psychology* devoted to the topic of psychiatric euthanasia.[5]

Sally Burgess and Keith Hawton, both psychiatrists at the Warneford Hospital, Oxford, first describe a case that became well-known as the Chabot case. This raises in acute form the issue of a doctor's conforming to the wishes of his patient. Dr Chabot worked in the Netherlands for an organization that supported assisted suicide, because he had learnt that they were finding it hard to recruit psychiatrists. The usual attitude of psychiatrists was one of complete opposition towards helping patients who wanted to end their lives. In 1991 Dr Chabot was visited by a Mrs Bosscher who said she was determined to die, and sought help to do so. She was in her fifties and in good physical health. She had been the victim of physical violence at the hands of her husband, an alcoholic, whom she had divorced many years before. She had two sons around whom her life revolved. The elder had committed suicide; the younger had quite recently died of cancer. On the night that her younger son died she had tried but failed to kill herself. Her determination to die was unwavering, and she wanted not to fail in her second attempt. The paradox of the case begins at this point. The fact that she consulted a psychiatrist might argue that she believed herself to be mentally ill. After all, if she decides to consult a psychiatrist, it is probably the patient herself who has concluded that there is 'something wrong with her', that she is 'ill' or at least 'not well'. Whether or not she has a disease that can be diagnosed and named is for the doctor to decide. On the other hand, more probably, she thought a psychiatrist the most likely doctor to help her achieve her aim, since her sufferings were not physical.

Dr Chabot examined Mrs Bosscher and found no evidence of any kind of mental illness, not even depression 'that would have responded to drugs', as he put it. Nevertheless he tried to persuade her to take anti-depressant drugs, and he also offered her a place in a therapeutic community; but she refused these offers, saying that all she wanted was to be able to kill herself successfully. He consulted two other psychiatrists and a GP, though they did not actually examine Mrs Bosscher. Dr Chabot decided that she was mentally competent, was suffering unbearably, and seriously wanted to die, for good reason. So he gave her a lethal draught in the presence of a friend. Charges were brought against him, but were dismissed by two courts. The case then came to the supreme court as a test case for psychiatric euthanasia. Dr Chabot was found guilty of unlawful killing, not because he had actively encouraged Mrs Bosscher to kill herself, but on the grounds that he had not caused her to be examined by any other doctor before doing so. But he was not punished, and was allowed to continue to practise. This perhaps tells us more about the chaotic condition of the law in the Netherlands at the time (for doctors who carried out euthanasia then did not know whether they would be prosecuted or not, nor whether, if prosecuted, they would be penalized) than about the moral judgment of the case, but it is worth considering it a bit further nonetheless.

For here is a case where a desire to die was considered rational, so irremediable was the unhappiness of the patient. She was not terminally ill, indeed she was not deemed to be ill at all, either physically or mentally. But it was thought certain that she would try again to kill herself, sooner or later, and the psychiatrist concluded that his normal duty to prevent suicide was overridden by the conviction that if he did not help her she would die after more suffering and in worse circumstances than those that he could provide for her. However it is a case that does not fit the evidence given by Dr Legemaate to the Select Committee. He said that psychiatric euthanasia might sometimes be carried out in the case of a patient, who, like Philip Graham, was severely mentally ill. He said nothing of a patient who was not mentally ill but who was simply rationally determined to die, there being no value left in her life from her point of view, and who wanted not only to kill herself, but to be enabled to die efficiently. Many doctors and nurses, and indeed farmers and vets who have access to drugs or poison, have killed themselves in the past. And many people have privately asked for help from their retired medical friends so that they could store up a collection of drugs for future use if they found life intolerable. (This humane practice is no longer possible; retired doctors may no longer sign prescriptions.) The suffering of Mrs Bosscher was thought by her doctor to be intolerable and many people would agree with him. But most who did agree would hope, however unrealistically, that she might learn to bear it, and find something in her life to value, so different is our attitude towards mental as opposed to physical suffering.

Suicide is not usually as easy as it was for Philip Graham, with his access to and experience with guns. The question is not whether unbearable mental suffering is ever a justification for suicide, but whether it can ever justify the provision of assistance for someone else who might not be able to bring it off unaided. We admit to feeling uneasy about the Chabot case. This is not because Mrs Bosscher was not terminally ill; we have argued that, in any future legislation, the closeness of death should not be considered a relevant factor, and that the prospect of years of suffering may be worse for a patient than the prospect of only months or weeks. The source of the unease is the indeterminate nature of the concepts of mental suffering, depression, and mental illness itself. Because they are inherently equivocal, there is always the danger that these concepts may be distorted or inappropriately deployed. There can be no doubt that Mrs Bosscher had had a horrible life, and that she sincerely believed that death was her only remedy. But should Dr Chabot have encouraged her in that belief? In the ordinary non-clinical sense she was depressed, and literally desperate. Dr Chabot thought that anti-depressant drugs would not help her (though he offered them), presumably because they could do nothing to change her circumstances. She had a lot to be, in the ordinary sense, depressed about. She refused treatment, as a patient has a right to do. But should he then have left her to make another attempt to kill herself? It seems that his motive for not doing so was simple compassion. Once again the problem is how to incorporate compassion into the law.

The next case is in some ways less problematic and it certainly fits better with Dr Legemaate's evidence about current practice in the Netherlands. It is that of an English woman in her thirties, Edwina, diagnosed as schizophrenic, and a long-standing psychiatric patient. She had several times been admitted to hospital with psychotic symptoms such as delusions, which had abated when she was in hospital under supervised medication. She also suffered from depression; and she particularly hated and reacted badly to hospital. When she was in hospital she became extremely distressed, constantly injuring herself and attempting suicide. But out of hospital she led a wretched life. She lived alone, her curtains always drawn, seeing nobody except the social worker allocated to 'care' for her in the community. She was unable or unwilling to maintain her medication or look after herself properly. She repeatedly said to her social worker that she wanted to be helped to die, since there seemed no other way out of her sufferings. She had a dismal quality of life, without any pleasure.

In the Netherlands, she would probably be one of the few candidates for psychiatric euthanasia. In Belgium, too, she might have been given euthanasia, for which, under the Act on Euthanasia 2002, the test is that the patient should be in a 'futile medical condition of constant and unbearable physical or mental suffering that cannot be alleviated'. This seems to cover her condition well enough, and she would probably gladly have settled for a lethal dose administered by a doctor.

In the UK, she would either be admitted to hospital against her will (as she had been several times) or continue to try to live outside until she either injured herself or someone else, perhaps fatally, in obedience to a delusive choice or imperative; or she would simply die of starvation or neglect. She is an example of someone for whom 'care in the community' is pitifully inadequate.

There is no doubt that Edwina, unlike Mrs Bosscher, suffered from a mental illness, or more than one, that could be diagnosed and named; and this made her case less problematic in at least one respect. If an illness affects a patient in more or less predictable ways, and if its symptoms (for instance the belief that one's thoughts have been inserted into one's head from outside) are common symptoms of the illness, then it must often be relatively easy to find more than one psychiatrist to agree on a diagnosis, even if the particular details of, say, the delusions experienced by the patient are unique. This being so, the risks attached to compulsory treatment are fewer (though we should never forget the political use that was made of compulsory treatment in psychiatric hospitals in the old USSR). In Edwina's case we can be sure that she was ill; and we can also be sure that if she did not go into hospital she would lead a miserable life. But in hospital her life would be just as miserable, or more so. Her position, like Mrs Bosscher's or indeed Philip Graham's, is literally without hope. She has what may well be an incurable disease. How then would we judge the psychiatrist who at least told her what she had to do to kill herself and put drugs at her disposal?

We return here to what is the central issue in this kind of case. Many people would say that a settled wish to die is the result of depression. Depression is an illness that can be treated and some-times cured or alleviated. Moreover depression is a mental illness; and mental illness is generally held to impair the judgment; so Edwina's declaration of her fixed wish to die cannot be given weight. A psychiatrist is a doctor whose duty must be always to treat and try to alleviate the sufferings of his patients who are ill; so it seems obvi-ous that he must not, instead, kill one of his patients or encourage her to kill herself.

But suppose that, as seems clear in Edwina's case, her illness will not be cured and that she will suffer from it as long as she lives. It is arguable that a law could be so drafted and so hedged about by safeguards that in such cases of identifiable and incurable mental illness, where the patient wished to die and repeatedly attempted to kill herself, assisting her to fulfil her wish might be lawful. It is not enough to say that, because she is mentally ill, her expressed wishes must be disregarded, when it is obvious both that she is suffering and that she can find no way out of her misery without help. Her suffering is not a mere sick fancy. It is an insult to write it off as such.

But to argue in this way is to rely heavily on the possible accuracy of a diagnosis (and a prognosis) of a mental illness. And, as we have already noticed, concepts in this field tend to be confused, and therefore unsafe. Society is not good at understanding, treating, or curing the mentally sick, and there is less than unanimity among psychiatrists. There is no such thing as palliative care in the field (for of course people like Edwina are chronically, not terminally, ill). Before we could set about changing the law to permit assisted suicide, we would need to understand a great deal more and be more sure in our classification of mental illness.

It is to be hoped that in the future we may learn more about mental illnesses and whether or not they can be cured, whether by drugs or conversation. We may learn better to distinguish illness from personality disorders which, we are told, cannot be treated at all. (If this is so, might not education have some part to play in mitigating them?) In the mean time, it is not surprising that, even in the climate of opinion in the Netherlands, and under their liberal legislature, it is hard to find a psychiatrist willing to practise euthanasia or assisted suicide on the mentally ill. Elsewhere in the world it is virtually impossible to envisage it at the present time. Even the right to refuse treatment is only a small step towards the right to be helped to end a life that is intolerable to the person who lives it. But we must not forget the suffering involved, even if legislation is unable, yet, to alleviate it.

# 4  Neonates

In the preceding chapters, we considered the central case of those people who, being mentally competent, express a serious wish to die. It is largely for their sake that campaigners for change want euthanasia or assisted suicide to be legalized in certain strictly controlled circumstances. But the question of legalized euthanasia arises also in the case of those who, for various reasons, cannot ask to die, but in whose best interests it may be argued that they should not continue to live. One such category is that of infants, new-born babies who are either extremely premature or who, even if the pregnancy is carried to term, are born with very serious disabilities and are unlikely to live long, or whose quality of life, if they do live, is likely to be very low. Here there is of course no question either of assisted suicide or of voluntary euthanasia. Someone else has to decide whether they should live or die. If death is ever to be the deliberate outcome, it will be non-voluntary euthanasia, generally regarded as the most indefensible form of death, practised only by intolerable tyrants, and to be avoided at all costs. According to one legal analyst, deliberately letting an infant die 'represents the only large-scale instance of involuntary euthanasia now being practised by the medical profession, at a time when most physicians and the public retain strong opposition to involuntary euthanasia in other circumstances'.[1] Things have changed since the 1970s and doctors are both more open and less inclined to take decisions of life or death on their own. But it is impossible to deny that any debate about euthanasia must take into account the practice of allowing neonates to die.

In the USA the first case of euthanasia for the new-born to hit the world headlines in modern times was that of Baby Doe, a case that had serious consequences. Baby Doe was born in 1982 in Bloomington Hospital, Indiana. He was born with Down's Syndrome. But he also suffered from an incomplete oesophagus, a defect not confined to Down's Syndrome babies, but more common among them. Unless he was soon operated on to reconstruct the passage from mouth to stomach, an operation that has a good chance of success, he would never be able to take food or drink by mouth, and would have to be artificially fed throughout his life or to die without nutrition or hydration. Dr Owens, the obstetrician in charge of the birth, noticed the condition of the baby and called in two paediatricians to consult on what should be done. The hospital where the baby was born did not have the equipment to carry out surgery to reconstruct the oesophagus, and the two paediatricians recommended that the baby be immediately transferred to the Riley Hospital in Indianapolis where surgery could take place. Dr Owens, on the other hand, recommended that Baby Doe remain at Bloomington to be cared for and kept comfortable but not fed intravenously, until his inevitable death. At this stage Mr and Mrs Doe were told of the conflicting recommendations of the doctors and the three doctors talked to the parents. The parents decided that they did not want the baby to live. Mr Doe was a teacher. He had some experience of

Down's Syndrome and argued that, even if surgery were successful, the quality of the baby's life in the future would be minimal. (He may also have found it impossible to reconcile himself to a child who could not shine academically. We do not know.) He argued that it would be in the best interests both of the baby and of his existing siblings that he should be allowed to die.

However, the management of Bloomington Hospital, including the welfare officers, questioned the decision and took the case to the local County Court, to be decided by a judge. This judge ruled in favour of the parents and Dr Owens. The welfare officers accepted the judgment, and were not prepared to appeal against it; but the county prosecutor then stepped in and asked a different judge to order intravenous feeding, so that the baby would be kept alive at least for a time, until further judicial opinion might be sought. This second judge refused to overturn the ruling of the first judge. The prosecutor's office nevertheless, still not satisfied, went to the Indiana State Supreme Court to ask for intervention to cause surgery to be carried out. This court, by a narrow majority, decided not to overrule the decision of the lower court. Despite all this, and despite the wishes of the parents, five days after the birth of Baby Doe, a member of the prosecutor's office flew to Washington, DC, seeking intervention by the United States Supreme Court to cause the surgery to be carried out. While he was on his journey the baby died.

This sorry story immediately became hot news, with furious editorials in both the *New York Times* and the *Washington Post*. To have allowed Baby Doe to die was seen as an infringement of the rights of disabled citizens. Section 504 of the 1973 Rehabilitation Act laid down that no recipient of federal funding might withhold from handicapped citizens (as the disabled were then known), simply because they were handicapped, any benefit or service that would be provided for people without handicaps. And it is true that, if Baby Doe had not suffered from Down's Syndrome, his parents would certainly have consented to his removal to Indianapolis for repair to his defective oesophagus.

President Reagan at once sent a memorandum to the Attorney General which concluded with the words 'I support Federal Laws prohibiting discrimination against the handicapped, and remain determined that such laws will be vigorously enforced.' Section 504 of the 1973 Act had been intended originally to include people with disabilities within the protection afforded to other minority groups, specifically blacks and women, from infringement of their human rights by the denial of generally available benefits or services. Now it was being invoked for a different purpose, the medical treatment of defective new-born babies. But there was nothing in the wording of the section to rule out such an extension of scope. Consequently notices were sent out to nearly 7,000 hospitals throughout the US, making it clear to administrators that federal funding would be cut off if they withheld from a handicapped infant nutritional sustenance or medical or surgical intervention to correct a life-threatening condition, if the withholding was based on the fact that the infant was handicapped. The notice, as it stood, entailed that, however severe the disability of the baby, the efforts made to preserve his life must be as strenuous as those that would be made to preserve the life of a non-disabled baby with a similar, separate malfunction. Moreover the notice, which had to be prominently displayed in all parts of a hospital where babies were treated, invited 'any person having knowledge that a handicapped infant is being discriminated against' to get in touch with the authorities via a special hotline that had been set up to deal with cases of discrimination, and pass on the names of doctors for possible prose-cution under the Act. Paediatricians understandably felt themselves to be under constant threat of prosecution when they had to make life or death decisions about severely defective neonates, the kinds of decisions that have always had to be made and with which they were sadly and increasingly familiar.

When the American Academy of Paediatrics contested the notice in court, it became clear that, despite its wording, the notice was intended to deal only with cases broadly similar to that of Baby Doe. Babies with Down's Syndrome have always been capable of survival if they are free from other malfunctions and, as they grow up, some of them are only quite moderately 'handicapped'. It was therefore easy to see how they might fall foul of section 504 if they were not treated for a reversible condition, for which babies without their disability would be treated. When challenged about children born with more severe disabilities, such as those born without a brain or intestines, the judge seemed to have no difficulty in excluding them from the provisions of the notice. The spokesman for the Department of Health and Human Services said to the paediatricians 'When you talk about a baby born without a brain, I suspect you meant an ancephalic child and we would not attempt to interfere with anyone dealing with that child. We think it should be given loving attention and would expect it to expire in a short time.' This suggests that cases that are really desperate will tend to be resolved without much difficulty, however much grief and sorrow is involved. The medical opinion of the hopelessness of the case will be accepted and the baby will be allowed to die.[2]

Among the difficult cases are those where the baby can survive, and where the question may not be how to reconcile the parents to its death, but how to reconcile them to its continued life. This was apparently the situation of Baby Doe. For, if a baby can survive, the issue is one of the quality of its life; and if it is decided that the quality of life will be so poor that death is preferable, then even if the baby is 'allowed to die' (and not actually be killed) its death will come about by the deliberate withholding or withdrawing of treatment, and this cannot be described otherwise than as non-voluntary euthanasia.

The question whether such euthanasia is ever justifiable, and, if so, whether it should be legalized in some situations, has become increasingly urgent, as babies have been born alive more and more prematurely, and more is known of the probability of severe disability for those extremely premature babies who are kept alive.

In the opinion of those who regard human life, whatever its quality or duration, as intrinsically and overridingly valuable, whether the living is an adult or a baby (or indeed a foetus or embryo), euthanasia should never be a defensible option. But there is a lack of consistency even here. A Working Party of the Nuffield Council on Bioethics has published a report[3] recommending that in some circumstances new-born babies should not be kept alive, but should be given 'comfort care' only and allowed to die. And this recommendation was endorsed by the official spokesman of the Church of England, which hitherto appeared to uphold the doctrine of the sanctity of human life. (Moreover, even more surprisingly, this spokesman said that, in considering whether a particular baby should live or die, the question of scarce resources that might be spent on futile attempts to keep it alive should be taken into account.)

The issue is this: today, premature infants born at twenty-four weeks gestation or even earlier and of very low birth weight, who, in the past, even if they had been born alive, would not have been viable, and those, whether premature or not, who are severely disabled at birth, may be saved, kept alive, and perhaps repeatedly resuscitated, as a result of sophisticated technology. Not long ago such infants would certainly have died soon after birth. Who should now have the authority to decide whether to keep them alive, or how and when to allow them to die?

More than twenty years ago, Dr A. Whitehead wrote

neonatal intensive care units have the ability to prolong the lives of infants with profound neurological abnormalities, including some who will never enjoy independent meaningful lives. Furthermore, neonatal intensive care is an expensive and rare resource which is sometimes denied to viable infants because of shortage of nurses and equipment. Against this background, many paediatricians have practised selection in applying high-technology life-supporting techniques.

That is, they have consigned some babies to die.[4]

Two of the considerations that have determined whether the baby is to live are here mentioned by Dr Whitehead: that of the quality of life predicted for him and that of the possible waste of resources from which other less disabled babies could benefit but of which they may be deprived in a situation of scarcity. Both these issues must be considered by the medical team, and both are part of medical responsibility. But of course the parents of a new-born baby are those most closely involved; and it seems to many people, and even to many doctors, intuitively obvious that theirs must be the decision as to whether the doctors should try every possible means to keep the baby alive, and for how long they should keep trying. Many people regard as outrageous the suggestion that a doctor might override the parents' wishes, and insist on withdrawing treatment from their baby, or decide not to intervene if the baby suffers a further relapse, let alone that this insistence should be based on financial considerations.

Before the days of high technology, when many more births took place at home, a doctor and a midwife attending a birth might make an instant decision on the first issue. They might see at once that a profoundly disabled baby was not going to survive for long, or might never lead a life that was worth living and might withhold immediate treatment that they might otherwise give (or might even quietly smother the baby), telling the mother that it had died in the course of birth, and comforting her as best they could. Prompt euthanasia, they might believe, would save the baby and his parents much suffering. Such paternalism is simply unthinkable today, if only because, in hospital, obstetric work is carried out by teams, all of whom may have some share in decision-making, and where decisions on resuscitation and intensive care have often to be made immediately. Moreover, there is a general assumption that doctors will be open with their patients and, as we have seen, that patients, or in this case their parents, should as far as possible decide what is to be done.

There is no going back; and it is true that in the old days doctors used to exercise immense power for which they could not be held to account. Yet we do not believe that one should entirely deride paternalism. After all, people consult their doctors, or depend on their services whether in childbirth or sickness, when they are themselves, in the nature of the case, relatively helpless. Often they feel precisely the need, if not for 'doctor's orders', then at least for medical advice, on the assumption that they themselves lack the relevant knowledge. If someone has just given birth to a severely disabled baby, or one with a precarious hold on life, she suffers not only from ignorance but from profound shock and distress. It is not wrong, in our opinion, that she should turn to her doctor for his medical experience, advice, and support. Some people argue that it is precisely because parents in this situation are so vulnerable that doctors should avoid paternalism. The vulnerable are easy to manipulate, even to exploit. That is what 'vulnerability' is. Doctors, according to this argument, have a duty, faced with this situation, to insist that parents exercise autonomy and make their own decisions as to whether the baby should live. But it may be psychologically or morally impossible for a parent to decide that treatment should be withdrawn or withheld from their baby. They may be unable to face the responsibility for what they see as a decision to cause the baby's death. Even assurances that it would not be their decision, but the underlying condition of the baby, that caused his death would not remove their guilt or self-reproach. In an article entitled 'Has the Emphasis on Autonomy gone too far?'[5] John J. Paris *et al.* suggest, taking their cue from Dostoevsky's *Brothers Karamazov*, that often individual choice or autonomy is not a right to be exercised but a burden to be shunned. Where a baby is desperately ill, parents' wishes may be complex; they may wish above all that their baby was not in the state he is in; they may wish that he be relieved of his suffering; and they may wish therefore that treatment be withdrawn, but that they should not be the ones who have to authorize its withdrawal. In the 'medical narrative', they argue, where a decision must be made whether a baby should begin or continue in intensive care, 'the best outcome from the perspective of those participating in the decision is one in which it is not clear who really made the decision, or even if one was being made'. We agree that this is the best outcome; and it is perhaps most likely to be achieved, as we have already suggested, where a baby is dramatically defective. If the baby is lacking some crucial organ, or is suffering from intercranial bleeding, for example, the decision to let it die, though tragic, will not generally be difficult and, once the parents understand the situation, will seem inevitable. 'We loved our baby but nothing could have saved him' may be their response. For in such cases it is clear that if the baby were to be kept alive artificially it would have no hope of even a conscious let alone a normal life. No medical or surgical intervention could remedy its condition.

The difficulties increase where a decision must be made on the probable qualities of a baby's life if he does survive, which, as we saw, was the case with Baby Doe. There are those who may think that Mr Doe grasped too readily at his son's defective oesophagus to insist that he be allowed to die, and point to the fact that the life of a Down's Syndrome child may be worthwhile and enjoyable for the child himself, even though his capacity is limited. Moreover there are frequent testimonies to the ability of whole families to love such a child and benefit from having him among their number. Such a life as his, they argue, should not be deliberately thrown away. However, it would be generally conceded that there are great difficulties in making judgements about the quality of someone else's life even in such cases as this. First, the severity of the effects of Down's Syndrome vary greatly, and it is impossible to tell at birth how severely affected a child will be. Secondly, while it used to be the case that those who were affected tended to die fairly young, usually succumbing to some infection, now, with antibiotics and other drugs available, they may well live until they are 50 or 60 years old. Many parents dread the idea of a disabled child outliving them, or living on when they are no longer able to look after him; and someone who has been an amiable and affectionate child, as Down's Syndrome children usually are, may become an aggressive, unmanageable, and unhappy adult. In the 1980s, Mr Doe would not have known this; but today his decision would be even more difficult. Equally, there is great variation among parents and other family members in their ability to live with the disability of their child.

The case of Charlotte Wyatt in the UK sadly illustrates this. Charlotte was born in 2004 at twenty-six weeks gestation, weighing about 458g (not much over 1lb). She was severely brain-damaged, and it was believed, even by her parents, that she was unlikely to live for more than a few months. However, they prayed for a miracle and asserted that she 'was not ready to die', though she did not respond to stimulation and seemed to experience nothing but pain. She stopped breathing several times and each time was given ventilation to resuscitate her. Later in 2004 the child's parents went to court in an attempt to overrule the doctors' decision that, if their baby should stop breathing again, she should not be reventilated. They argued that their love would support her, and that she must be given every chance to live. On the grounds of the child's best interests, the judge ruled that, in spite of the parents' claim to know intuitively what was and was not tolerable for their baby, the medical opinion must prevail that her best interests lay in being kept comfortable, and being allowed to die if she stopped breathing. In the event, she continued to live without further ventilation and at last the parents were allowed to take her home. But four years later, Charlotte being still alive but entirely helpless from the brain-damage she had suffered, they separated; the strain of looking after the child had been too much for them. The child is still alive at the time of writing, but with no prospect of ever leaving hospital again.

When cases arise where doctors and parents cannot agree about the future treatment of their child and the matter is taken to court, it generally happens that the judge finds in favour of the doctors.

**Neonates**

Once judges have accepted medical evidence that there is little or no prospect of a child's improving and that further treatment would be not only futile but burdensome and distressing, they understandably decide that the child must be allowed to die, sympathetic though they may be towards the distress of the parents. It is true that in 2006 a judge found against the doctors.[6] In this case he did so on the grounds that, although the child would not improve, according to his parents he did show some cognitive function, and he enjoyed their company, watching television, and hearing songs. The quality of his life was thus judged according to the criterion of whether or not he was capable of experiencing pleasure. This was a judgment that showed sympathy both for the parents and the child. But it was unusual.

Sheila McLean, Professor of Law and Ethics in Medicine at the University of Glasgow, has argued that the present system of decision-making in neonatal medicine is deeply flawed.[7] She writes

Doubtless it was simpler when babies with severe disability had no prospect of remaining alive. No ethical code was needed to reach conclusions. Ultimately nature decided for us. But this is no longer the case.... Like it or not, decisions are made on a daily basis that some infants should not be kept alive. No one school of thought seems to have convinced parents, doctors and the law. The result is uncertainty, inconsistency and confusion.

She argues that doctors have too much power in deciding whether to treat an infant or let it die, even if they can no longer hide their actions or failures to act under the cloak of the privacy of home delivery. For, Professor McLean argues, even where doctors and parents disagree and the issue falls to be settled in court, judges are unduly influenced by the authority of doctors and their tendency to support other members of their profession. There was a notorious case in the UK in 1981 (even before Baby Doe) when the parents of Down's Syndrome baby, John Pearson, did not want him to live, though, unlike Baby Doe, he apparently suffered from no other defect. Dr Leonard Arthur issued the order 'nursing care only'; and the baby would presumably have been given water only until he died. But Dr Arthur, probably on compassionate grounds, ordered a massive dose of sedatives as well, and the baby died almost immediately. A member of the hospital staff reported the matter to a pro-life organization who took it to the police, and Dr Arthur was charged with murder (a charge later changed to 'attempted murder'). At the trial several eminent medical witnesses were called to testify that Dr Arthur's treatment of the baby fell within acceptable professional standards. In his summing up, the judge addressed the jury in these words: 'I imagine that you will think long and hard before concluding that eminent doctors have evolved standards that amount to committing a crime'. Dr. Arthur was accordingly acquitted on the basis of the authority and consistency of the medical evidence.[8]

Professor McLean, quoting this case, concludes that leaving decisions about infant euthanasia to doctors, even if they consult with parents, and even if the case comes to court, is not safe. Her suggested solution is that there should be new and tightly drawn legislative guidelines which the judiciary can apply, if need be, with total independence of 'expert witnesses'. They may hear both clinical and parental evidence, but the final decision-making must be open, impartial, and above all consistent. The greater the power of technology to keep infants alive, the more necessary such judicial guidelines become.

The Report of the Nuffield Council on Bioethics, to which I referred above, a closely argued and compassionate document, considers the question whether new legislation is needed to govern medical practice in allowing defective neonates to die. They conclude, like Professor McLean, that what are needed are firm guidelines. They consider the possibility of legislation regarding euthanasia that would cover only decisions relating to new-born babies, but reject this, largely because it could not offer the certainty and predictability of outcome that would presumably be its aim, and because it would remove an essential element of judgement around particular circumstances that must inform any decision to be agreed between doctors and parents. Recognizing the difficulty in determining what is in the best interests of the baby, and especially in assessing the pain and distress that a neonate may feel, they nevertheless conclude that the present legal framework within which agreement must be sought between doctors and parents as to the best interests of the child is the best that can be found.

Among the new guidelines that they propose are those laying down what should be normal practice in instituting intensive care for babies who are born very prematurely. They recommend that there should not be any attempt to keep alive a baby born before twenty-two weeks gestation; at twenty-four weeks and beyond, normal practice should be that invasive intensive care will be started; at twenty-three weeks, where predictions of the outcome are most difficult, precedence should be given to the wishes of the parents, and to the judgement of experienced paediatricians. It seems to us that having such guidelines in place, well-known to doctors, nurses, and parents, will make agreement on treatment easier.

Already, in good hospitals, there exists trust between parents and doctors, whose overriding aim is that there should be agreement about the best interests of the baby, so that decisions about withholding or withdrawing treatment may be reached imperceptibly and without confrontation. This is genuinely a matter of trust, where a mother believes absolutely that the doctor will do all that he can for her, her baby, and the rest of her family, and taking a case before a court should almost always be avoidable.

It is largely on the grounds that it would erode this essential trust that the Nuffield Working Party turns down any suggestion that, if a baby is to die, it should be given a lethal injection, rather than having its treatment withdrawn or withheld and given 'comfort treatment' only until it dies. Apart from this pragmatic objection, they leave open the question whether what they call 'active euthanasia' (otherwise 'killing') can ever be justified. Some members of the committee apparently thought that it could. But there is a suggestion in the report (para. 6.38, p. 105) that this could be justified for an adult only if that adult had asked for it; and that, because babies cannot make their wishes known, a baby must never be killed, but only allowed to die. The taboo against killing is extremely powerful.

In paragraphs 2.38 and 6.36, bringing about the death of a baby who was suffering extreme pain that was impossible to alleviate otherwise is justified by the doctors' friend, the doctrine of double effect. They say: 'The Working Party takes the view that, provided treatment is guided by the best interests of a baby, and has been agreed in the joint decision-making process, potentially life-shortening but pain-relieving treatments are morally acceptable.'[9]

We will say more about this argument, and about the distinction between killing and letting die when discussing the more general medical attitudes towards euthanasia (Chapter 8 below). In the context of the non-voluntary euthanasia of infants, it seems to us that the Nuffield Working Party, whose report was intended as a contribution to good practice not to philosophy, has done well. If the guidelines are drawn up according to their recommendations, some of the uncertainty of the present situation, especially with regard to very premature babies, will be removed, and things will in future be easier both for doctors and, marginally, for parents, though nothing can take away their sorrow.

# 5 Incompetent Adults

We turn now to other cases of non-voluntary euthanasia, a kind of mercy killing where a decision may be made to bring about the death of a patient, although the patient has not, and could not have, asked for it, at the time when the decision was made. It is important to include the qualification 'at the time when the decision was made', for there are some cases where a patient, though mentally incompetent at the time of death, himself made a declaration in advance, while he was still competent, in which he formally made his wishes known about his treatment in case, when he approached death, he had become unable to make his own decisions. These advance decisions will be discussed first.

The purpose of an advance decision (also known as an advance directive or a living will) is to give a patient who is suffering from, say, dementia, or who is in a permanent vegetative state the same right to refuse treatment as is enjoyed by a competent patient. As the law stands in the UK, no one may be given assistance to die through an advance directive; nor can they demand any specific treatment, for example to be kept alive until they die naturally. All they can ask is that, if they fall ill when they can no longer make their own decisions, treatment shall be withheld (or withdrawn if it has already been started, in an emergency). In the past, at least in the UK, the status of an advance decision, even if it had been formally drawn up and signed before witnesses, was uncertain. We have been told, for example, in personal correspondence, of a case where a woman, Mrs K, had her explicit instructions disregarded, because the doctor in charge of her case believed that as long as a patient was alive every effort must be made to keep her alive, whatever the quality of her life. Mrs K, who had led an extremely active life, and was a highly successful and intelligent woman, had become unable to live by herself when she was in her eighties because she had lost her sight, and was becoming increasingly frail. Her daughter found her a place in a nursing home, and before Mrs K took up the place, she made an advance decision, with the help of her solicitor, requiring that she should not be given treatment if she should fall ill, but should be kept comfortable until she died. She made it clear that this was her settled wish, and would remain her wish, whatever her mental state in the future. The nursing home held a copy of the document, and agreed that its contents would be honoured. However one day Mrs K contracted pneumonia, and the doctor who looked after all the patients in the home ordered that a course of antibiotics should be started that evening. When her daughter heard this, she went at once to the home to try to prevent it happening. At first the nurse on night duty said that she must obey the doctor's orders; but she was reluctantly persuaded to wait for twenty-four hours, in which time Mrs K's daughter found another doctor who, when he heard the situation, agreed to take Mrs K onto his list. He came round to examine her the following morning and ordered that there should be no treatment, but only nursing care. Mrs K lost consciousness within a few hours and died in the evening, with both her daughters at her bedside, as she would have wished.

This story would have been even more shocking if the treatment proposed by the first doctor had been, not drugs, but intrusive and potentially distressing intervention, such as Mrs K had specifically ruled out in her decision. But it is shocking still, because the doctor was putting his moral scruples (he was a member of a Christian doctors' group, which held as a matter of principle that every possible measure must be taken to preserve life) before the express wishes of his patient, who was no longer in a position to refuse treatment. (As it happens, Mrs K and her daughters were all Roman Catholics, but found no difficulty in holding that in the circumstances it was rational, and not immoral, to prefer death to life.) The question whether a doctor may put his own conscience above the wishes of his patient will be discussed in more detail later.

In England, the Mental Capacity Act, which came into force at the beginning of 2007, should make it more difficult for a doctor to disregard the earlier expressed wishes of a patient at the end of life. The Act starts with a statement of the principles that lie behind its provisions, one of which is that any decision taken for or on behalf of someone who lacks capacity must be taken in that person's best interest. And section 4 lays down that whoever is determining what is in the best interest of an incapacitated person must consider that person's past and present feelings, and in particular any relevant written statement made by him when he had capacity. And later, in section 24, it specifies what is to count as a valid form of advance decision.

But this still falls short of making even a properly drawn up advance decision legally binding. For section 25 states that an advance decision shall not be applicable to a particular form of treatment, if it is reasonable to believe that circumstances have changed in a way that the author of the decision could not have known, and which would have affected his decision if he had anticipated them. It could perhaps be argued by Mrs K's first doctor that treatment for pneumonia had changed in ways that she could not have known, and that therefore he was justified in disregarding her decision. But of course what she wanted was to be allowed to use pneumonia as her 'friend', as it used to be called, bringing about a merciful death for the old when their life had ceased to be a pleasure to them. She did not want the pneumonia to be treated, however new and revolutionary the treatment.

Nevertheless, it is to be hoped that, despite considerable opposition to treating advance decisions as absolutely binding, the Act will bring about a change in the general climate of opinion, so that such decisions may be taken more seriously in determining what is to happen to the incompetent at the end of life, and also that more people may come to make such decisions, as a matter of routine.

The USA has been ahead of the UK in this matter. In the USA, in general, doctors and judges seem to give more weight to the probable wishes of the incompetent patient in determining her best interest. In 1989, the parents of a young woman, Nancy Cruzan, were told by the Supreme Court in Missouri that they had no right to require that her life-support machine should be switched off, although she had been declared to be in a permanent vegetative state, and had no hope of recovery. The parents appealed to the Supreme Court of the USA and lost their appeal. In his judgment, Justice Rehnquist asserted, instead, the right of the State of Missouri to insist that she continue to live, out of respect for the intrinsic value of human life. He argued that it was the duty of the state to protect a life as long as it exists, whatever its quality, and even if continuing to live is contrary to the patient's best interest. (Justice Scalia, concurring, went further. He said that a state had the right to prevent death, and it need not honour an advance decision, if it has decided that letting someone die is an insult to life's sanctity.) However, surprisingly, Justice Rehnquist laid down that, if proof could be found that Nancy Cruzan had seriously and formally declared that, if she should ever be reduced to the condition she was now in, she would wish life support to be withdrawn, then it should be withdrawn. Her parents asserted that she had made such a statement, but they could produce no proof; and so she had to live on. With continued effort, and the advice of many lawyers, the parents managed to produce 'clear and convincing evidence' of her wishes, as the court had demanded, and, taking the case to a lower court, won permission for the machines to be switched off. This time no one took the case to a higher court, and after seven years in a permanent vegetative state, she died.

As a result of Nancy Cruzan's case it was generally recognized that if someone had made clear what they would wish to happen to them in a situation like hers, the state was bound to honour that wish. Several states immediately changed their own laws to take this into account, and by now every US state has provision for advance decisions in some form. As early as 1990 a law was adopted by Congress that required any hospital in receipt of federal funding to inform all patients who come into hospital for treatment of the law regarding advance decisions, and the correct form in which to record such a decision if they want to be sure that they are not kept alive in the case that, during their stay in hospital, they should become incompetent; and this information is given to literally all patients, even those who come in to have the most routine procedures carried out. In the USA an advance decision thus now trumps any other judgment of what is in a patient's interest, and it also trumps any general argument based on the sanctity of life.

We hope that we may move towards this position in the UK. Suppose someone suffering from dementia and who had made an advance decision that if she should begin to suffer the failure of some organ, say the kidneys, no heroic measures should be taken to keep her alive; and suppose further that a new means of restoring function to the kidneys had been found, of which she would not have known when she made the decision, it might be natural for a conscientious doctor to think that he should give her the latest and best treatment. On the other hand, if she survived as a result of the treatment she would still be as demented as she had been when she grew ill; and it was from this state of dementia that she wanted to be released. If a new cure had been found for dementia, it would doubtless be different.

At any rate, it should be possible, through GPs' surgeries and health centres to educate people about advance decisions, so that they are far more routinely drawn up than is the case at present. And so gradually it would become the normal expectation not only of the aged, but of the young and healthy that they would not be allowed to linger on in the sorry situation of a Nancy Cruzan. Moreover, as the organization Dignity in Dying argues, there are new summary care records being developed as part of the NHS Care Records Service; and it would be easy to include in such records the existence of an advance decision, so that it would be less likely that a patient's decision should fail to be known when the crisis came.

However, even in the USA, decisions about allowing incompetent patients to die do not always involve speculation about what they would have wanted had they foreseen their present situation. For example there was a notorious case, carried to its conclusion in

2005 in the glare of publicity, that of the American woman, Terri Schiavo, in Florida. She had suffered irreversible brain damage and had been kept alive by artificial feeding and hydration for many years. Her husband wanted the tubes removed. He thought of her as to all intents and purposes already dead. He said 'Terri died fifteen years ago. It's time for her to be with the Lord.' Her parents, on the other hand, thought of her as alive and well. They paid no attention to the opinion of the doctors who had examined her that she would never recover brain-function. They ran a campaign website to try to save her life, on which they declared 'Terri is a purposefully interactive, alert, curious, lovely young woman who lives with a very serious disability'. To allow her to die would be not only to take a life wrongfully, but to discriminate against the disabled. No one would after all think of killing her if it were not for her disability. The case came to court and the judges ruled that disability discrimination was irrelevant to the case (surely rightly), and that the tubes should be removed. George W. Bush, the President, rushed back from his Easter holiday to insist that they be replaced, in the name of religion (though, judging by his words, Mr Schiavo was also a believer). But he failed to overrule the judiciary. The tubes were not replaced and Terri died within a few days.[1]

In the UK, the legal situation concerning patients who, like Nancy Cruzan, were in a permanent vegetative state was clarified in 1993, when the House of Lords Appellate Court confirmed a judgment that it was lawful for a young man called Anthony Bland to be allowed to die.[2] In 1989, Bland had been injured in the Hillsborough football stadium disaster, his lungs crushed so that his brain was deprived of oxygen, and though his other injuries were treated successfully, he was declared after a year to be in a permanent vegetative state (PVS). This meant that, though his eyes were open, he saw nothing; indeed he had no experiences of any kind. With careful nursing, attention to bedsores and hygiene, and with artificial nutrition and hydration, he could have lived for many years (he was only 19 at the time of the accident), but his parents wanted him to be allowed to die. However the Airedale Hospital Trust under whose care he was were, understandably, uncertain of the law, and feared that they could be found guilty of corporate murder if they deliberately removed the tubes that supplied him with nutrition (he did not need ventilation, his lungs having recovered completely, so that he could breathe unaided). The case attracted enormous publicity, many people never having heard of PVS before. At first the press concentrated on the question whether it was possible that he might recover, and there was a series of stories of people miraculously 'coming round' after years in a coma. But the evidence of the severity of his brain-damage was made clear, and the question then became that which the appellate judges had to settle, namely could deliberately causing Bland's death be lawful? There was no question of his being terminally ill, nor of his suffering being intolerable, since he did not suffer at all, being completely unaware of anything either within himself or in the world around him. His parents were not asking that he be put out of his misery; it was they who were miserable, not he. It was the futility and pointlessness of his condition and the possible length of its duration that made them so. They could perhaps come to accept the idea that he was dead, but not the idea that he was alive yet to all intents and purposes dead. They argued that, given his character, he would prefer to die than to live in this condition, if he had been able to form a preference. But they did not attempt to prove this to the judges. The judges relied mostly on the concept of his best interests, in coming to the decision that it was lawful for the tubes to be removed so that he might die.

But even here there was difficulty. 'Best interests' is not an unambiguous concept. Lord Justice Mustill, one of the appellate judges, argued that one could not defend the judgment on the grounds that it was in Bland's best interest to die. He said: 'he does not know what is happening to his body, and cannot be affronted by it; he does not know of his family's continuing sorrow. The distressing truth which must not be shirked is that [discontinuing life support] is not in the best interests of Anthony Bland for he has no best interests of any kind.' This suggests that if someone is unconscious and is not going to regain consciousness nothing is either in his best or his worst interests; it does not matter what happens to him, from his point of view. But Ronald Dworkin in his book, *Life's Dominion*, distinguishes between two kinds of 'interest', 'experiential' interest and 'critical' interest.[3] The former is what you feel at any given moment to be in your interest, for example, to be given food if you are hungry; but the latter is more abstract. It takes into account what you think of, or once would have thought of, as a 'good life'. Your 'critical interests', seem to suggest an Aristotelian concept of a good life, involving not how you feel at the moment, whether you are enjoying yourself or not at any particular time, but whether, surveying your life as a whole, you feel satisfied with how it is and will be. Aristotle quotes Solon's saying: 'call no man happy until he is dead'.[4] It is only a whole life that can be judged happy or unhappy. Your interest, on this view, includes how you would like to be thought of after you are dead; it includes, that is to say, an idea of the narrative of your life. In this sense it must be argued that for Bland it would not have been in his interests to stay alive, with his family gradually forgetting the person he used to be and remembering only the pitiful figure he now was. But in any case the judges were not moved solely by consideration of Bland's best interest. They placed considerable weight on the distinction between withdrawing treatment (in his case held to include artificial hydration and nutrition) and actively intervening to cause death, between act and omission. We shall return to this highly dubious argument, beloved of doctors as well as judges, when we come to consider the medical attitudes towards assisted dying, in Chapter 8.

Yet another argument by which the judges defended their decision that Bland be allowed to die was that, if Bland had been conscious and competent, he could have chosen to have treatment withdrawn; and their decision granted him the same right as he would have had if he had been competent, (and which he might also have been able to exercise if he had made an advance decision, which of course he had not).

These last two justifications led to an enormous debate. Both of them turned on the inclusion of artificial nutrition and hydration being deemed to be treatment. It was argued strongly, especially by the nursing profession, that the withdrawal of treatment did not include the supplying of these basic needs to a patient. Supplying a patient with food and water was the fundamental duty of care owed by nurses and doctors to everyone, however hopeless their condition, and their professional integrity would not allow that this be withdrawn. It ran totally against the professional and humanitarian training that nurses had been given to refuse food and drink to anyone, no matter how it was delivered. They suggested that if feeding by nasogastric tube were to be deemed treatment, then so would feeding someone with a specially designed cup or even a teaspoon.

Obviously there was another way in which Bland's life could have been brought to an end, and that was by giving him a lethal injection. But this would have been euthanasia by any definition, and to legitimize euthanasia would have involved changing the law, which was not contemplated at the first hearing. The case therefore went up to the Court of Appeal, and, with great difficulty the appellate judges decided that artificial feeding and hydration is a form of treatment and therefore might be withdrawn from Bland without fear of prosecution.

Some Law Lords were not entirely happy with the result. One of them, Lord Justice Browne-Wilkinson, questioned why it was morally right to allow a patient to die slowly by withdrawing nutrition, and therefore lawful to do so in certain circumstances, and morally wrong to bring about his death by lethal injection, which remains unlawful in all circumstances. He could find no satisfactory answer to his own question.

However, the Bland judgment stands; and it became a matter of central importance in the debates on the Mental Capacity Bill. The issue was whether or not an advance decision demanding that treatment be withdrawn if a patient should become ill when incompetent should be taken to include the withdrawal of nutrition and hydration. There were those in both Houses of Parliament who argued passionately that no advance decision could entitle, or compel, nurses and doctors to withhold food and water, or allow another human being to die of starvation and thirst. The debate was extremely emotional, terrible stories being told of helpless and demented patients being starved to death, or otherwise dying of neglect.

But 'Bland' has not been overturned by the Mental Capacity Act. In opposing an amendment to the Bill that would have made it unlawful to withdraw artificial nutrition and hydration from incompetent patients, Baroness Murphy, a geriatric psychiatrist of great experience, argued that to speak of allowing patients to die of starvation and thirst was misleading. She said this:

Artificial nutrition and hydration are invasive medical treatments that fall clearly into the category of treatment that would be included if an individual said that they wished to refuse life-saving interventions. They involve the insertion of a nasogastric tube, which is not pleasant at all, or the intravenous infusions of artificial nutrients and chemicals. The paraphernalia restrict movement, and the process requires extensive monitoring. It is uncomfortable and very often distressing…The whole procedure is burdensome. While the burdens are generally acceptable to people during a temporary acute illness or during a period after an operation from which one is hoping to recover, they are rarely justified as a long-term form of care when someone is approaching the end of life during a fatal illness…If the individual is at home the question never arises. If they are being cared for by the family, tubes and drips are not put in. The possibility arises only when somebody goes into hospital and receives unnecessary interventions. Having written a letter to express my wish that, in the event of my becoming incapacitated, I do not wish to have life-saving treatments, I have assumed that my statement includes those burdensome treatments.

And she ended:

Comfort is all. The many patients with dementia for whom I have cared have two serious physical problems at the very end of life. The first is their skin care and the comfortable disposition of their body; and the second is oral care and the hydration of the mouth. It is possible to maintain somebody's hydration without all the artificial intravenous paraphernalia. When we are near death, we all crave the right touch rather than the right food.[5]

For those patients who are incompetent and who have not made an advance decision, or in cases where there is doubt about the validity or applicability of the decision, the Mental Capacity Act now allows that the Court of Protection, which formerly had powers to decide only matters concerned with finance, may determine matters of health and social well-being as well. Moreover, someone may be granted Lasting Power of Attorney who may decide on the basis of the best interest of the patient whether treatment may be withdrawn. And if there is no one who has this power, the Court of Protection may appoint a deputy to act on his behalf.

Nevertheless, though the Mental Capacity Act is to be welcomed, in so far as it clarifies the situations in which decisions may be made not to prolong the life of someone who is incompetent, such decisions will apply only to an incompetent patient who becomes acutely ill while incompetent. There remain thousands of patients who, as the opponents of the Act alleged, are simply neglected and die because of this neglect. Neither the Mental Capacity Act, nor of course any Bill that sought to legitimize assisted suicide or euthanasia for those who wanted to die, can do anything for these patients. There is a terrible description by the author, Alan Bennett, of some of the old women who shared a room with his mother, all of them suffering from dementia.[6] There was a high turnover of these women in the room, because they soon died of malnutrition. The 'carers' in the nursing home were mostly young and untrained, and very much overworked. They put down a tray of food, sometimes even out of reach, but had no time to help the patients eat it, slow spoonful by spoonful. The tray was collected whether the food had been eaten or not; and so they wasted away. Mrs Bennett survived because she had always been very fond of food, and somehow kept her appetite. As Baroness Murphy said, in the speech from which I have already quoted, such neglect is a matter of poor standards of care, and is a problem that needs urgently to be addressed, but not in the context of the Mental Capacity Act.

**Incompetent Adults**

Contemplating the wretched lives of patients with dementia who do not have the luck to need artificial nutrition and hydration, who are conscious and capable of swallowing, and whose numbers are increasing every year, we may feel despair. They are allowed to die, many of them, by a slow and horrible death, far from the 'good death' or the 'death with dignity' that euthanasia would afford them. Many of their relatives, if there are any, must long for them to die. But many of them have no relatives, or none that visit them. Even if palliative care for the dying were far more widely available than it is, they would not qualify for it; for they are not, or not necessarily, terminally ill, or suffering acutely. What is to be done? This is a question to which, as far as we can see, society can at present supply no answer. But it must be faced, as we become an increasingly aged population.

# 6 Human Life is Sacred

In his evidence to the House of Lords Select Committee on the Assisted Dying for the Terminally Ill Bill, Professor Jonathan Glover, of the Centre of Medical Law and Ethics at King's College London, said in his opening remarks: 'The central argument against the Bill at the level of moral principle [is] the sanctity of human life, sometimes defended on religious grounds, but sometimes supported for quite secular reasons.'[1] This remark can be generalized to cover not just Lord Joffe's Bill, but any proposal for assisted dying of whatever kind. This chapter is an attempt to analyse and assess the principle of the sanctity of life.

In 1965, Lord Devlin enunciated the principle thus:

A murderer who acts only upon the consent, and maybe the request, of his victim is no menace to others, but he does threaten one of the great moral principles upon which society is based, that is the sanctity of human life. There is only one explanation of what has hitherto been accepted as the basis for the criminal law and that is that there are certain...moral principles which society requires to be observed and the breach of them is an offence not merely against the person who is injured but against society as a whole.[2]

## Human Life is Sacred

Devlin was here arguing in favour of the continued criminal-
ization of homosexual acts between consenting males; murder
was cited only as an analogy. But the underlying argument is
the same. No matter what compassion, or desire, may dictate,
society and the rule of law rest on certain agreed moral principles which form, as he elsewhere says, the 'cement' that holds
society together. Society will collapse without this adhesive material. Devlin's views of homosexuality may seem to us, now, eccen-
tric; but his view on the sanctity of human life would be widely
accepted.

Yet, though Jonathan Glover is certainly right to say that the principle of sanctity may be invoked in both a religious and a secular
context, the idea of the sacred has strongly religious origins. Every
religion, from the earliest known time, has had sacred objects, the
desecration or violation of which has been held to be punishable if
not by man, then by the gods themselves. There have been sacred
animals, such as cows or cats, sacred rituals, sacred places, groves,
mountains or the ark of the covenant; and of course there are sacred
texts. The sacred induces awe as well as respect; sacred things must
be kept safe at all costs; even to mock them is blasphemy and may
call down the wrath of heaven.

Not all religions have held human life to be sacred in this sense.
Even Abraham was prepared to sacrifice his only son, Isaac, at the
yet more sacred command of God; and the God of Israel was by no
means the only god to demand human sacrifice. However, the most
unequivocal statement of the sanctity of life in recent times is to be
found in the written evidence presented to the Select Committee on
Lord Joffe's Bill by the archbishops of Canterbury and Westminster
and the Chief Rabbi .

The Memorandum by the Office of the Chief Rabbi said this:

Jewish tradition places at its centre the sanctity of life, viewing life as a precious gift from God, not something we can dispose of at will. Indeed, the value of human life is absolute and not relative to factors such as age and health. The commandment of the preservation of human life is a central one in Jewish teaching. Furthermore the Ten Commandments emphasise the prohibition of murder; in addition there is a strict prohibition against suicide in the Jewish legal code. Therefore Judaism regards the value of human life as non-negotiable and insists that it cannot be compromised.

And the passage goes on:

As an eminent authority on Jewish law and ethics, Rabbi J. D. Bleich has stated, in summarizing the Jewish view on euthanasia: 'Any positive act designed to hasten the death of the patient is equated with murder in Jewish law, even if the death is hastened only by a matter of moments. No matter how laudable the intentions of the person performing an act of mercy-killing may be, his deed constitutes an act of homicide.'... In summary, Judaism cannot purchase relief from pain and misery at the cost of life itself.

This is the view expounded by the previous Chief Rabbi of England, Lord Jakobovits, who argued that life was infinitely valuable; and since infinity is indivisible, it follows that every bit of life, however small, and however miserable, is equally infinitely valuable, so that it can make no difference whether one shortens life by seventy years or seventy seconds, nor whether the victim is young or old, healthy or dying.[3] (This is the absolutist position, embraced by orthodox Judaism, but not by reformists. They hold that life is of value almost beyond everything, but yet is not an absolute value, for its value must be determined by the circumstances in which the life is being lived.)

## Human Life is Sacred

The submission of the Christian bishops, though less detailed and perhaps marginally less dogmatic than that of the orthodox Chief Rabbi, is equally definite about the origin of their fundamental opposition to any attempt to legalize assisted suicide. They wrote: 'The arguments presented in this submission grow out of our belief that God himself has given to humankind the gift of life. As such, it is to be revered and cherished.' The God-given is sacred.

As for the Muslim community, though they did not submit written evidence, Dr Khalid Hameed, as their spokesman, gave oral evidence to the Select Committee. He said that he would not accept requests or instructions to end the life of one of his patients because it is against his beliefs. 'If I had to give advice to a fellow Muslim patient, I would advise them strongly that we were both believers and we would both end up in hell. If the patient is another denomination, I would end up in hell and I do not know about him. Best of luck.'[4] This we suppose is a religious argument for the sanctity of life, though rather a startling one. But it does at least serve to emphasize the fact that arguments derived from the specific religious dogma embraced by whoever is opposing assisted suicide or euthanasia need not have much relevance to those who do not share the faith in question. Dr Hameed was speaking, however, as a medical doctor, not as a cleric; and the substance of his evidence was based on his fear of the social consequences of a change in the law, a version of the slippery slope argument that will be examined in the next chapter.

It is indeed noticeable that most of those who oppose a change in the law on grounds of the sanctity of life in the religious sense, even if they start from the statement that life is God's gift, and as such must be taken away only by God, move thereafter to a more pragmatic argument, based on the supposed social consequences of permitting assisted death. Strictly, they should not need this move; for a theologian, or an adherent of a faith that asserts life as a gift from the creator, the theological argument should be enough: there is no danger of sliding down to the bottom of a slope if you never allow yourself even to contemplate approaching its top. But the fact that most theologians do make this move raises the question whether by the 'sanctity of life' they mean more than that human life is a very important value. If this is all they mean, then whether any other value may sometimes override it must be decided by the circumstances, the view put forward by the reformist rabbis.

In fact, even if one believes that life is a gift from God, it does not necessarily follow that death must also come from the hand of God. There are Christians, Jews, and Muslims who believe that some human beings commit crimes which render them deserving of death, and that it is only of the innocent that it can be said that their life is a gift from God which no one is entitled to take away. For, after all, most gifts are thought, once given, to belong to and be the responsibility of the person who received the gift. The donor loses all rights over what he gave, though he may sometimes attach conditions to it, as is the case with trusts set up for specific purposes. Perhaps the religious argument would be more plausible, even for believers, if the emphasis were more on the suggestion that life is held in trust for God's purposes than that it is a gift. Then the justification of capital punishment, for those who defend it, would be that the murderer has shown himself unworthy of the trust and must surrender it.

In any case, it has usually been assumed, even by those who assert the sanctity of life, that a man is justified in killing another in self-defence, presumably on the grounds that the aggressor is no longer innocent. It is for this reason, too, that the problem of what is a just war, and how a just war ought to be conducted, has become so central to morality; for in the conditions of modern warfare huge numbers of casualties will be innocent, in any intelligible sense of the word. Guilt by association is hardly enough to destroy the innocence of children.

So it seems that there must always be exceptions to the assertion of the absolute and overriding value of human life in general, however crucial, both to morality and the law, must be its protection in normal circumstances. But of course the subject of this book is life in circumstances that, even if not uncommon, can hardly be described as normal.

However this may be, it is less than illuminating, and perhaps positively obfuscating, to discuss 'life' as an abstract concept, a kind of Platonic Idea or Form, identifiably common to all the things that are alive, and itself possessed of an intrinsic value. Even Buddhists, who believe that all lives form a kind of continuum and that the taking of life is to be avoided as far as possible, nevertheless distinguish between human life and that of other organisms; and in the Judaeo-Christian tradition, it is only human life that has unique value.

There is, after all, no such stuff as life, no vital fluid, poured out into different vessels, the bodies of human beings and other animals and plants. There are only living organisms, each one with a developing life to lead, a potential story; and this is as true of molluscs as of men. But it is to human organisms, developed to have consciousness, imagination, and the ability to form their own aspirations and pursue their own interests that we ascribe unique value. It is of human beings that we should say they are supremely valuable. Life is not what is 'sacred', only lives, each lived by some individual person. It is upon this value that the law of murder is founded.

This value is not dependent upon a belief in any god or gods; indeed it is fundamental to non-religious people, who may indeed describe themselves as 'humanist', as well as to the religious. So what do religious believers add when they speak of life as sacred, or as a gift from God? They add, of course, the authority that they ascribe to the language of religion, the authority of a sacred text, held to contain the commands of God, and the authority of a whole culture based, in the English-speaking world, largely on the Judaeo-Christian tradition. And there is no doubt that this tradition has been enormously influential in the formation both of morality and the law. But religion is a man-made phenomenon, as is morality itself, and the law. They have grown up together, but have for centuries been conceptually separable, separated by philosophers such as David Hume, who was sardonically sceptical of all religious revelation, and even by the more respectful Kant, who held that religious language must necessarily be metaphorical: to believe otherwise would be plain anthropomorphism.

For those brought up within the tradition of a particular religion, it may often be true that religious language is the most expressive language to use, in formulating a principle that is in fact a principle of morality or of politics. For example, in justifying the spending of public money on the education of severely mentally disabled children, who will never be able to contribute to the economy, it may be an expressive short-hand to say 'they are all God's children'. But this is a way of stating a principle of equality, or under the present law of claiming for them a human right.

It is probably pointless to ask which came first, the morality or the religion. What is true is that the metaphor of God's children, though significant for those brought up within a religious tradition, may be barely intelligible to someone brought up with no concept of any religion at all. The sanctity of human life, if this means that life is a gift from God, or is held in trust for God's purposes, is equally a short-hand that has sense for those who believe or even half-believe in God (for it is an over-simplification to suppose that everyone is either an atheist or a believer). But for the rest it has to be translated into a moral and a legal principle, that each human being is to be valued and his life protected, unless some other value is, in particular circumstances, to be given priority. So in some parts of the USA justice is thought to be a higher value, where someone has committed murder, and justice demands that the murderer himself be killed; or in time of war, defence of a soldier's country may demand that he sacrifice his life. The 'sanctity' of human life may be a real and living concept for those who believe in a living God; but for others, it is, like much in the language, a left-over, suggestive still, but insubstantial, like the fragrance of cigar smoke left behind by someone who has walked away.

If this is so, though it is true, as Jonathan Glover said, that the sanctity of life is often invoked in a secular context, it perhaps should not be, or not as if it added anything to the moral and legal truth that would be universally admitted, namely that human lives are valuable, and that no one must be deprived of life unless there are compelling higher values that can justify such an act. To quote Glover again: 'Secular accounts of the sanctity-of-life view will be highly implausible to those who see human life not as a good in itself, but rather as a precondition for something else. It will be an unattractive position to all those who, for example, see life in a permanent coma as in no way preferable to death.'5

Far-reaching questions are raised by the confusing of moral with religious arguments in the matter of the value of human lives. It is obvious that believers, of whatever faith, are perfectly entitled to derive moral and political principles from the tenets of their belief-system, but this does not entitle them to commit offences against the law, unless they are prepared to face criminal charges. The rule of law governs everyone, whatever religion they adhere to, and whether or not they profess faith in any religion. It is more difficult to answer the question whether religious belief should have any particular influence over legislation. The fact that in England at least there is an established church and the existence of the Bishops' Bench in the House of Lords may seem to give the Christian religion an undue influence in legislative matters. Lord Joffe, in a debate about the rights of people who profess no faith, certainly blamed the defeat of his last attempt to introduce his Bill on assisted suicide for the terminally ill on the influence of Christian dogma—not, however the dogma of the established church, but primarily on that of Roman Catholicism. He called attention to the huge campaigning efforts against the Bill, initiated by the Roman Catholic archbishop of Cardiff, and pointed to, among other things, large numbers of identical lobbying letters from all parts of the country. He quoted an article opposing the Bill in the *Catholic Times*, written by Father Marsden, and illustrated by a photograph of twenty-four children murdered by the Nazis,[6] and said: 'Self-evidently that had nothing to do with the Bill and it was, in my view, a disgrace and obscene'. He went on to raise the question whether it is right that church leaders should mount a campaign with the intention of imposing their beliefs on the majority of the population who do not share those beliefs.[7] This is certainly an important question. But it is of interest that the offending article

## Human Life is Sacred

relied not on a belief in the sanctity of life, or its being God's sole prerogative to end it, but first and foremost on the belief that the passage of Lord Joffe's Bill would lead to the killing of children on grounds of dogma. It was noted above that most of those who deploy the dogmatic or theological argument against any form of euthanasia soon turn to a quite different argument, supposedly empirical, and based on the consequences that will flow from a change in the law. Such was Father Marsden's reasoning. So it is time to turn to this kind of opposition to euthanasia, the dreaded slippery slope.

But before doing so, it is perhaps proper to end this chapter by stating our conviction that those who hope that the law may one day be changed are totally convinced that members of society have an obligation to one another, which imposes on them the duty to save human lives where they can, and to do nothing to lower the quality of the lives of their fellows. This is a duty laid especially upon the medical professions, but it belongs to us all. The question is whether a blind reverence for the preservation of life at all costs, and however low its quality, may not sometimes stand in the way of this duty.

# 7 The Slippery Slope

In the last chapter we considered the a priori argument against any change in the law of murder that would permit euthanasia or assisted suicide. The sanctity of human life argument purports to be absolute, depending for its force not on any consideration of consequences, but on the intrinsic wrongness of deliberately depriving someone of life. We argued that most people who claim to base their opposition on this argument, though they genuinely believe that human life is of the utmost value, nevertheless go on to reinforce it by pointing to the evil consequences to society that would follow from allowing any weakening of the taboo that forbids the deliberate taking of life. They move from the a priori to the empirical, almost without noticing that they are doing so. Perhaps they are uneasily aware that society allows some exceptions to the sanctity principle, for instance in accepting killing another in self-defence, and so they turn to a social or consequentialist argument to be on safer ground. One member of the Select Committee that considered Lord Joffe's Bill, however, did make the distinction between the two kinds of argument quite clearly. In the debate on the committee's report, he said

## The Slippery Slope

The sanctity of life argument—perhaps I may call it that—is not my reason for opposing this legislation. As legislators our religious beliefs are bound to inform our deliberations, but our overriding concern and responsibility should be to consider the best interests of society as a whole; that is, for those with religious beliefs and those without.[1]

This is an extremely important distinction. It suggests that, regardless of private conviction, whether religious or based on compassion, in determining public policy, those who have responsibility to make laws or change them must rely on broadly utilitarian arguments, that is, they must take account not of the intrinsic nature of the act that would be permitted under a new law, but of the consequences that such acts would have for society as a whole. An argument relying on probable consequences is an empirical argument, appealing to supposed facts rather than theory, faith, or dogma. If one is to oppose such an argument one must question whether the facts are indeed as they are portrayed. Will the consequences necessarily be harmful for society? This particular speaker explained his fear: 'My reason for believing that this legislation would not be in the best interests of society is based on a genuine concern about the fundamental change in attitudes and belief regarding the end of life that I am convinced would result from a change in the law.' This is the very heart of the slippery slope argument. If you once allow one exception to the law that forbids the deliberate ending of a human life, then inevitably further exceptions will be made, and the supreme value that we accord to human life, whether expressed in terms of its 'sanctity' or otherwise, will, as a matter of fact, be eroded. Once that process has begun, there will be no stopping it: it will lead us into nameless horrors.

There is no doubt that this form of argument has an immense appeal to the imagination, and is deployed in many different contexts, wherever a change in a law is proposed, or an exception to a rule contemplated. The argument can be set out formally as follows: it may seem at first sight all right to do x (whatever x may be); but x will inevitably lead to y and y in turn to z; everyone agrees that z is intolerable, therefore one must not do x. X, which at first appeared relatively harmless, even desirable, has now become wrong on account of the 'inevitable' consequences that will flow from it.

The inevitability of the descent down the slope is not a matter of logical necessity. It is not that accepting euthanasia for competent patients who request it actually entails the acceptance of euthanasia for other patients. If we accept that all men are mortal, and that Socrates is a man, then we must inevitably accept that Socrates is mortal, if we are to be consistent. We must inevitably assent to the conclusion if we assent to the premises; it is a matter of strict entailment. We can formalize the argument, and thus lift it out of the realm of the empirical world: 'If all x is y, and z is x, then z is y'. To hold that a change in the law would 'inevitably' lead to dire consequences, on the other hand, is to make a prediction about the world of experience. It is based on our knowledge of human nature; on the way things tend to go.

To see whether such arguments are generally valid, we need to consider different versions of the slippery slope. There are situations in which a slippery slope argument, though not a matter of logic, is still very powerful. If someone is trying to give up smoking, and says 'There can be no harm in just one cigarette', his friend may argue: 'One cigarette wouldn't harm you, But one will inevitably lead to another, and you will soon end up smoking as much as you did before. I advise you against it.' Given what we know about nicotine addiction, this forecast is well-founded, and his friend would be sensible to take his advice, unless the one cigarette he proposed to smoke were the last cigarette in the world. But this narrowly conceived slope has no relevance to euthanasia. Even though a doctor from the Netherlands is reported to have said that administering a lethal injection to his patients became easier as he became more accustomed to it, this cannot be thought to have turned him into an addict who could not stop himself from killing. That might be a just description of the notorious Dr Shipman; but the existence of a law against killing one's patients plainly made no difference to him. No one who opposes the proposal to change the law believes that, if the law were changed, we should end up killing people for pleasure, as Dr Shipman apparently did.

A different form of the slippery slope argument might be named the uncertainty principle. It is sometimes argued that if a law contains terms that are impossible to define precisely, then inevitably that law will become more permissive than was at first proposed. This form of the argument was sometimes used in opposition to Lord Joffe's Bills. It was held that, though they were supposed to permit assisted death only for the terminally ill, and only for those who were experiencing unbearable suffering, since neither of these two terms was capable of precise definition, there could be no clear limit to the number of patients who might be helped to die. There is no discernible difference between someone who is likely to die in four weeks time and someone who will die in five. Nor is there a discernible difference between suffering that is very bad and suffering that is intolerable. So the permission for assistance cannot be properly restricted. This is a version of a paradox known to the Greeks as sorites. It turned on the definition of a pile of sand.

There is no doubt that one grain of sand is not a pile. And there is no discernible difference between one grain of sand and two; but if you go on adding sand, grain by grain, in the end you have a pile. However, there is no single moment when you can claim to have a pile. A pile of sand is a hopelessly indefinite entity, and one that would be abhorrent to lawyers.

In some cases, it is possible to overcome this kind of uncertainty in a law by fixing an arbitrary but precisely calculable limit. A speed limit is of this kind. And, to take another example, in the British Human Fertilization and Embryology Act of 1990, a limit was set on the time an embryo might be kept alive in the laboratory. It might be kept for fourteen days from the beginning of fertilization, after which time it would be a criminal offence to have a live embryo in your laboratory. This limit was often criticized at first, because there was, it was said, no discernible difference between an embryo of fourteen days, and one of fifteen, and yet a scientist became a criminal if he crossed this line even by an hour. This was said to be indefensibly arbitrary and, seeing this, people would disregard the law.

The limit of fourteen days was in fact not completely arbitrary, in that it corresponded more or less with an important stage in the maturing of an embryo, just as a thirty mile speed limit is not completely arbitrary; it is calculated according to the safe stopping time of motor vehicles. But the merit of the fourteen day limit was that it was precisely measurable, and therefore gave rise to the certainty that the law needs. It was a regulatory line, which had to be drawn somewhere, and once drawn was unambiguous. Indeed it has proved a useful line both in the clinical procedure of IVF and in research, and it remains as part of the revised embryology law.

## The Slippery Slope

The difficulty, in contrast, with 'terminal illness' and with 'unbearable suffering' is that they are intrinsically indefinite, the first because it refers to the future, and one cannot exactly predict the date of anyone's death; the second because tolerability or otherwise depends on the person who is suffering. We do not think that this constitutes an insuperable difficulty in the way of drafting a Bill that would permit assisted death in certain circumstances for someone competent who asked for it. But it must be admitted that the law does not like the open-ended.

It is perhaps worth noticing that the sorites or no discernible difference type of argument is sometimes held to be logical rather than empirical. For, it is said, it would logically inconsistent to accept one kind of action and reject another when there is no discernible difference between them. In accepting the first (say, using a fourteen day embryo for research) we are logically committed to accepting the second (using a fifteen day embryo) James Rachels puts it thus: 'Once a certain practice is accepted, from a logical point of view we are committed to accepting certain other practices as well since there are no good reasons for not going on to accept the additional practices once we have taken the all-important first step.' And he distinguishes this from the psychological form of the argument, that once the first step is taken people will in fact go on to further steps.[2] We do not accept that this is a matter of strict logic. It is rather that those who use the sorites form of the slippery slope argument are saying that, as a matter of human nature, if there is no discernible difference between X and Y, Y will come to be practised as well as X.

The most usual form of the slippery slope argument against the legalization of euthanasia is less precise than either of the two foregoing versions. Indeed, it is not very often that it is formulated otherwise than in the very general terms of the abuse that must inevitably follow from the passage of any such law. For example, in her admirable book, *The Right to Die*, Miriam Cosic recounts the story of the nine months during which the Northern Territory in Australia had a law permitting voluntary euthanasia, and the subsequent overturning of that law by federal government.[3] She quotes a vocal opponent of the Bill, Chris Wake, an Anglo-Catholic, but one who claimed that his opposition was not based on his religious belief. Of the debate in Darwin when the law was passed for the Northern Territory he is quoted as saying 'The rationale on which I proceeded [to oppose the Bill] had nothing to do with religion. This argument needs fighting on earth here and now, not in heaven, after.' And he went on: 'It's the socio-economic aspects of euthanasia being applied in Australia which frightens me to death because I think, in fact I *know*, it would be misused. And I haven't seen anything anywhere in the world ... that came within a cooee of ensuring that abuse would not occur.'[4]

It is true that any Bill, to have a chance of success, would have to contain safeguards against abuse; there would necessarily have to be conditions laid down on the face of the Bill, to ensure that the patient asking for euthanasia knew what he was asking, was competent to make decisions, and was not suffering from temporary depression that could be remedied. In the Netherlands, the doctor has to have known the patient for a specified length of time, in order that he can be sure of understanding his true wishes (though this condition is not always observed). In Lord Joffe's proposed Bills a psychiatrist had to see the patient; the request had, if at all possible, to be written and signed, and a fortnight had to elapse between the request and its execution. But none of these safeguards are sufficient to allay the fears of those who rely on the slippery slope argument.

## The Slippery Slope

It has to be remembered that all such arguments are speculative; what we are warned against is a hypothetical future that we are told will come about if the law is changed. The abortion law in the UK is often used as an analogy. When the Act was passed in 1967, it seemed that it contained enough safeguards to ensure that women could not just demand an abortion for convenience, or on a whim. They had to convince two doctors that their mental or physical health or that of their family was at risk if the pregnancy continued. But gradually the conditions have been relaxed, and the number of abortions has soared. However this analogy is by no means exact, if only because before 1967 abortion was already widely and increasingly carried out by 'back-street' practitioners, who caused many deaths. Indeed, part of the purpose of the new law was to bring this to an end by ensuring that abortions were performed only competently, and by those licensed to do so. There is a difference between attempting to control by regulation a practice that is widespread, increasingly in demand and dangerous, and attempting to permit a practice that will arguably never be widely in demand. We hold that the case against euthanasia must be defended separately, and not built on a doubtful analogy.

The difficulty lies in the fact that though the slippery slope argument is empirical, in that it is concerned with a predicted future 'on earth here and now', it is difficult, if not impossible, to produce evidence with which to support it. The National Council for Hospice and Specialist Palliative Care Services began the summary of their submission to the Select Committee by complaining that 'there is a dearth of methodologically robust research into the impact that Physician Assisted Dying would have in the UK'.[5] It is not surprising. We are here in the realm of guesswork, or at best of common assumptions about human nature.

So what are the abuses that the Australian, Chris Wake 'knew' would follow a change in the law? What is said to lie at the bottom of the slope varies according to the person or the group of people who deploy the argument.

One of the fears most commonly expressed is that, if assisted death were an option, patients in the last stages of their illness might have pressure put on them to ask for it, when it was not what they really wanted. It is not difficult to imagine feeling that one's children were getting impatient either for their inheritance or simply for relief from the burden of care, and that one had not so much a right to ask for death, as a duty to do so, now that it was lawful to provide it. There undoubtedly exist predatory or simply exhausted relatives. But it is insulting to those who ask to be allowed to die to assume that they are incapable of making a genuinely independent choice, free from influence. (Indeed, there are people so determined to confound their children, if they see them as vultures hovering over a hoped-for corpse, that their will to spite them by staying alive may outweigh their wish to escape their own pain).

In any case, to ask for death for the sake of one's children or other close relatives can be seen as an admirable thing to do, not in the least indicative of undue pressure, or pressure of any kind. Other kinds of altruism are generally thought worthy of praise. Why should one not admire this final altruistic act? And it would not be wholly altruistic: the desire to avoid squandering resources, or being a burden is combined, in the cases we are considering, with a sense that prolonging life is both futile and painful. It is idle to try to separate these motives. Part of what makes a patient's suffering intolerable may be the sense that he is ruining other people's lives. If he feels this keenly, and asks to be allowed to die, he is not a vulnerable victim, but a rational moral agent.

## The Slippery Slope

In those parts of the world where assisted dying has been made lawful, the first condition has been that the patient should formally ask for euthanasia or assisted suicide. However, the most powerfully emotive versions of the slippery slope argument have been those that foresee this condition somehow withering away with the passage of time, so that it will come about that the lives of those who have not asked to die will be deliberately ended. The deliberate ending of life would no longer be taboo, so anyone might be at risk. This seems to be the real fear expressed, for example, by Chris Wake whom we quoted above.

It is often suggested that the fear is borne out by what happens in the Netherlands, where it is said that at least a thousand deaths a year are brought about by non-voluntary euthanasia, where the patient has not asked to die, but a doctor has decided that it would be in his best interest to do so. This should officially be classed as murder, rather than euthanasia.[6] However, the figures, though often repeated, are not very reliable: in the first place, since non-voluntary euthanasia is illegal in the Netherlands, it is unsurprising that evidence of its occurrence is difficult to collect. Secondly, in the Netherlands such figures as there are include the withdrawing of treatment from very premature or damaged new-born babies. Thirdly, the safeguards included in the Netherlands euthanasia Act are not as stringent as those contained, for example, in the Death with Dignity Act in the State of Oregon. It is possible therefore that still more stringent legislation, if it could be drafted, would serve to block the descent down the slippery slope which leads to non-voluntary euthanasia. In her examination of the evidence supporting the claim that in the Netherlands society, or doctors and lawyers, have slid down the slope from voluntary to non-voluntary euthanasia, Dr Penney Lewis argues that there is no evidence that non-voluntary euthanasia has increased because of the legalization of the voluntary, nor is there evidence from Oregon or Belgium. One should not therefore rely on 'The Netherlands experience' as an argument against a change in the law.[7]

In any case, it is generally supposed that there are cases, and not only in the Netherlands, where doctors have assisted the death of patients who have not requested it when they, the doctors, have judged that the patient's suffering has gone on long enough. Some research carried out by Professor Clive Seale, Professor of Sociology at Brunel University, sought to establish the figures for non-voluntary euthanasia in the UK.[8] The answers to the questionnaire that he sent out showed that doctors were far more likely to ascribe the performance of such euthanasia to others than to themselves; but however unreliable the data, what emerged was that it is at least widely believed that cases of non-voluntary euthanasia do occur. In fact it is plausible to argue that the existence of a law on the statute book spelling out the conditions under which alone assisted dying was permissible would itself act as a block to prevent descent down the slope and would make it less likely rather than more that unlawful non-voluntary euthanasia would take place. For it would be easy to ascertain that the conditions and safeguards required in the law had not been satisfied in the case of a suspicious death.

We do not in fact need to rely on suspicion or dubious statistics to tell us that non-voluntary euthanasia occurs. For under this heading we may properly include cases such as that of Bland and Terri Schiavo (see Chapter 5). Here the justification for allowing the patients to die was that they would not recover any sort of cognitive function or capacity for enjoyment; that, though they did not suffer themselves, their meaningful life was over, and that their families (or, in the case of Schiavo, her husband) were suffering pointlessly. In his

## The Slippery Slope

book, *Aiming to Kill*, the Roman Catholic priest, Nigel Biggar distinguishes between 'biological' and 'responsible' life. Interestingly, it is only to the latter that he ascribes 'sanctity'. Where a patient has biological but no responsible life, either because he suffers from massive brain damage, or from such overwhelming pain that it requires analgesic palliation that is no less overwhelming, then it is morally right that he be allowed to die. This is his preliminary conclusion. However, at the end of his book, after considering the slippery slope argument, he overturns this preliminary finding. He writes:

The withdrawal of treatment [from a patient with PVS] rests on the judgement that human life that is forever bereft of the capacity for responsible life is not worth the costs of sustaining it; and here the costs are not those of the patient, who is beyond suffering, but the emotional burden borne by the family and the economic costs to the community. ... However, ... if we permit the withdrawal or withholding of treatment in the case of a patient with PVS because we consider this form of human life not worth sustaining, will we be able to draw a convincing line between this kind of case, where the lack of responsible life is more ambiguous?

And he goes on to quote from the BMA Guidance, published in 1999, which endorses the withholding or withdrawal of tube-delivered food and water not only from patients in PVS but also from other non-terminally ill patients such as those with dementia or serious stroke. And he concludes from this 'lack of discernible difference' argument (or 'not being able to draw a convincing line') that patients in PVS must be kept alive with artificial nutrition and hydration and the use of antibiotics to combat infection. He admits that this conclusion is paradoxical. For he recognizes that competent patients who are less badly off than those in PVS are entitled to refuse treatment and be allowed to die. He recognizes also that he himself, on a preliminary view, could find no moral objection to allowing such patients to die. But he comforts himself with the thought that 'extreme cases' should not dominate the argument, and that anyway they are few in number.[9] Here, then, is a slippery slope at the bottom of which is supposed to lie the killing of those patients who, while not necessarily in pain, nor suffering greatly, are judged to have a low quality of life. They have not asked to die, so their death is non-voluntary euthanasia.

It is usually this kind of slippery slope argument that is relied on by the numerous disabled groups who are violently opposed to a change in the law, though their opposition is not always very clearly argued. They feel themselves threatened by any attempt to legitimize assisted death, believing that such a law would become an instrument in the unfair discrimination against the disabled that they see in society at large. They suggest that, even were assisted death to be available only to the terminally ill, in the perception of the public there is no difference between severe disability and terminal illness; and, more important, it is assumed by the public that it is better to be dead than to live with a severe disability, especially one that is progressive. Therefore it will become acceptable to offer the option of death to the disabled, whether or not they have asked for it spontaneously. When a disabled person begins to feel that a doctor or nurse regards the quality of his life as very low, he may be inclined to go along with the judgement and accept an offer of death, even an implicit offer. This amounts to undue pressure, such as to invalidate his choice, even if he appears to have made one.

It is true that one should be cautious about judging the quality of other people's lives. And one must not confuse the value that someone attaches to his own life (or the quality he ascribes to it) with the value we think we would attach to such a life, if it were ours. Still less must we slip into thinking that a life of poor quality is somehow objectively 'valueless'. It is the value of the life as it is lived by the person, not any value that it has in someone else's eyes, that is crucial in determining whether he should go on living. But there is an enormous gap between a Tony Bland, one who is unable to ascribe any value whatever to his own life, and a disabled person who is conscious and capable of having experiences, pleasures as well as pains. There is a 'convincing line' to be drawn between them; and to fear a slippery slope here seems unnecessarily timid, if not paranoid.

Understandable as they are, the fears of the disabled appear to be misplaced. Recent evidence has shown that in both Oregon and the Netherlands rates of assisted dying show no evidence of heightened risk for several vulnerable groups, notably the disabled, the elderly, and those with psychiatric illness. Thus, where assisted dying is already legal there is no current evidence for the claim that legalized physician-assisted dying or euthanasia will have a disproportionate impact on patients in vulnerable groups and put these groups at risk of undue pressure to agree to end their lives.[10]

There is one more version of the slippery slope to be considered. People often say that if physician-assisted dying were permitted in any form whatever, the trust between patient and doctor would be fatally eroded. It is alleged that patients who are ill, especially if they are otherwise vulnerable through age or disability, fear to go into hospital, because they will never know whether the doctor is coming to their bedside to try to make them better or to kill them. It is perfectly true, as we acknowledged at the outset, that it is in a hospital setting that doctors have to make life or death decisions about patients. And no one could deny that there is something intrinsically frightening for most people about hospitals, full as they are of doctors and nurses about whom one knows nothing. On the other hand there are patients who when they realize that they have a condition that will be painful and may be terminal say that they believe their doctor will 'make it all right'. And by this they do not mean that the doctor will cure them, but that he will ensure that death, if it is to come, will not be too agonizing or long-drawn-out. As a matter of fact, it is more often members of the medical profession than their potential patients who use this form of the slippery slope argument; and the attitude of doctors to physician-assisted death is the subject of the following two chapters. What we have tried to do in this chapter is to suggest that the aim of legislators, if the law is to be changed, must be to block the slippery slope, or render it less slippery than is often supposed. It must be said in conclusion that some of the predicted consequences of a change in the law, though they might be horrible if they occurred, seem less threatening and certainly less inevitable than others.

# 8  Medical Views

The next two chapters will draw together a range of attitudes found among the medical and nursing professions in response to the complex issues at the end of patients' lives. We will examine the concepts of killing and letting die, the doctrine of double effect, futility, and the role of training and conscience.

In the next chapter we will look in greater clinical detail at assisted suicide, self-denial of food and fluids, and euthanasia, and assess the position of palliative sedation in the ethical spectrum. We will also explore the emotional effect on physicians of participating in the ending of life. We will finally summarize our own conclusions for appropriate measures now.

Doctors in general are of a conservative turn of mind when contemplating decisions involving their patients. Medicine is a discipline in which taking risks with patient welfare is almost never justified and doctors, even those trained to model their care on the latest evidence-based research, are not easily persuaded to change a long established policy. It is not surprising that the contemplation of such profoundly serious changes of practice as assisted suicide and euthanasia has led to controversy, disagreement, and fierce professional debate. Doctors are currently forbidden, like every other citizen, to end human life. There is no legal indulgence conferred by a medical or nursing qualification.

So what attitudes do these professionals express when discussing the interests of patients in grave distress who seek medical aid to end their lives? In medical ethics much discussion centres on the difference between 'killing' and 'letting die'. For many people it seems important to distinguish between killing and letting die and to prohibit the former while authorizing the latter in certain cases. In the past the distinction was sometimes, not very helpfully, referred to as that between 'active' and 'passive' euthanasia. In recent years, however, the distinction between killing and letting die has become blurred. For example, switching off a respiratory-support machine could be interpreted as actively terminating a patient's life. Alternatively this act may be seen as withdrawing the artificial means maintaining a life which is already unsustainable by the individual alone. In other words this act discontinues an artificial circulation in a patient who is actually already dead (letting die).

We would contend that there is no *morally* relevant difference between killing someone and allowing him to die. A well-known example cited in medical ethics describes two young men, each of whom want their 6-year-old cousin to die in order that they can gain a large inheritance. Smith drowns his cousin while the boy is taking a bath. Jones plans to drown his cousin, but as he enters the bathroom he sees the boy slip and hit his head: Jones stands by doing nothing while the boy drowns.

Smith killed his cousin: Jones merely allowed his cousin to die.[1] Both of these acts are clearly reprehensible but do demonstrate that the distinction between killing and letting die is *morally* irrelevant. Moreover, someone who starves another person to death is as guilty of murder as someone who poisons that person. The person who allows a fellow human being to die of hunger is as morally guilty as someone who acts to poison him. The difference lies in the more obvious and direct causal implications of the verb 'to kill'. Killing, like pushing or pulling, kicking or smashing, is manifestly doing something to produce a certain effect. John Stuart Mill insisted that a cause is not necessarily an 'active intervention'. The failure of the guards to patrol the walls may cause the fall of the city.[2] Yet people may still instinctively feel that failing to do something is less causal than killing them. It is less 'hands on'. It is after all doing nothing, and may therefore seem to be incapable of producing any effect. *Ex nihilo nihil fit*. Moreover, 'to kill' is a verb that contains a record of its own success. If I kill you, you are dead; whereas if I, say, fail to feed you, there is room for another event to come along either to save or to dispatch you. There is space for what the lawyers call *novus actus interveniens*.

A case that illustrates the medical abhorrence of active intervention to bring about death was that of a 40-year-old woman known only as Ms B. In 2001 she suffered a burst blood vessel in her neck and became totally paralysed. She was kept alive on a ventilator for a year, her brain unaffected. When the year was up, she asked that she might get someone to switch off the ventilator at a time of her choice, when she felt she had had enough. The hospital authorities refused, and one of the doctors involved was reported as saying: 'She is asking us to kill her, and this we would not like to do'. Ms B appealed to the courts, and a court was convened round her bed. The judge, Lady Butler-Sloss found that she was suffering from no mental incapacity, and that it would be lawful for the hospital to grant her request. They still repeated that they could not kill her, even if it would be a lawful act. So Ms B was moved to another,

## Medical Views

less squeamish hospital, where in due course she asked for the ventilator to be switched off and she died.[3]

Thus, doctors are profoundly suspicious of any action which may be classified as killing; and this is partly, we believe, because of the emotive violence contained within the very word 'killing'. This word carries with it images of battlefields or grisly car accidents. These images are far removed from the scene of calm, caring, easeful, and timely death that is the ideal we would all wish eventually for ourselves.

We could perhaps examine this medical suspicion further by substituting a more neutral term such as 'termination of life' rather than 'killing'. In discussing the concept of termination of life, doctors frequently protest that such an idea is against all their training and instinct. On closer examination, however, we may ask whether this is really true. Doctors are trained to care for their patients and support them both physically and emotionally to the best of their ability. The best interests of the patient are described as paramount. This implies that the best interests of the patient are of overriding importance in all circumstances, the problematic as well as the straightforward.

Doctors work intensively in a complex environment and are required to make value judgements in weighing up the pros and cons of virtually any medical management decision. Relevant weight is given to different aspects of the situation, both physical and emotional, before a plan of action is agreed with the patient. Thus doctors become practised at estimating values, mainly perhaps subconsciously. Value judgements may weigh in the balance, for instance, side-effects as against longevity, patient views as against those of their family, current discomfort as against future gain, possible damage to one organ as against benefit to another.

Furthermore doctors make life and death decisions in many circumstances. These value judgements are the most crucial, and are not infrequent. For example, should a patient with widespread advanced malignancy be resuscitated in the event of a cardiac arrest? What would the patient want in the circumstances: an easy exit or a long-drawn-out uncomfortable death? Patient views vary, but some undoubtedly would prefer to avoid more painkillers, constipation, drips, and enemas and be remembered by their family as the whole person they were before their disease undermined them.

Another example: should renal dialysis be commenced in a patient who already has other very severe medical problems likely to prove fatal in the near future? Renal dialysis is a very demanding form of therapy both for the patient and the staff, entailing as it does three times weekly connection of the circulation for many hours to a fixed dialysis machine. Not only may the burdens of this treatment outweigh the benefits for the individual but also another patient may be deprived of the potential for greater, more long-lasting benefit.

In either case, unless the doctor swiftly evaluates the situation, makes a decision, and acts promptly, the patient will die in the immediate future. Doctors therefore already make life and death decisions. Both the decisions we have used as examples are of course made against the background of a limited potential survival, in a sense decisions to let die sooner rather than (not too much) later. The two cases exemplify decisions involving letting patients die. Morally, however, it is highly arguable that there is little difference between allowing death to take place and actively terminating life. In moral terms doctors could find the distinction between these cases and euthanasia, both based as they are on judgements as to suffering and value of life, more difficult to draw than first appears.

## Medical Views

What view do the courts take of the distinction between killing and letting die? In the many medical cases which have come before the courts, where a doctor's action has resulted in death, the defence of double effect has been cited. The doctrine of double effect has a long history among Roman Catholic theorists as a moral defence for intervening during failing labour to save the life of the mother while sacrificing the life of the unborn child, or as a defence for killing someone in self-defence. The argument rests upon the moral acceptability of performing an act with the intention of doing good which nonetheless has an unintended, although foreseen, unwelcome consequence. A well recognized example involves the administration of a high dose of painkiller which is intended to relieve pain although it is realized that death is a possible, though not the intended, outcome. The doctrine thus assumes that it is possible to draw a clear distinction between what someone intends while actually carrying out a particular action, and what his intentions are towards the probable outcome of the actions he is performing. The law is accustomed to reaching conclusions about a defendant's momentary intention in acting, indeed the law of murder demands that such a distinction be drawn. Common sense is less certain. In any case, it is more realistic to describe the doctor's thinking when administering the painkiller as another instance of a value judgement: that it is more important, in the particular case, to relieve the patient's pain than to keep him alive.

In the medical context the doctrine of double effect was clearly articulated by Mr Justice Devlin (later Lord Devlin) when he summed up to the jury in the Bodkin Adams case. Dr Bodkin Adams, a general practitioner, was accused of murder by overdosing his elderly patient with morphine in order to benefit under her will. The argument has been that a dose of painkiller (morphine or diamorphine) which is required to control extremely severe pain in terminal patients may have the unintended consequence of terminating the life of that patient. However, this argument, which has held a central place in the defence of doctors accused of murder or manslaughter, carries somewhat less weight today. Previously when patients developed very severe illness such as cancer associated with a great deal of pain, strong painkillers such as 'the Brompton cocktail', morphine or diamorphine were administered intermittently (usually along with a bottle of Scotch) in order to relieve severe symptoms. More recently the development of palliative care as a specialty has facilitated the refinement of pain management in both choice and delivery of effective medication. It is now very possible in most cases for pain, even when severe, to be well controlled by the sustained administration of analgesia which just controls the person's symptoms (while still enabling the patient to remain alert and cognitively functional). The need for sudden, potentially life-threatening high-dose medication has largely been eliminated. Thus the argument that doctors need to deliver sudden increases in morphine or other drugs which risk ending life is now unlikely to persuade a court that the doctor was well intended. The doctrine of double effect is thus now likely to prove less persuasive.

Yet despite advances in palliative medicine, there remains a small proportion of patients in the last days and hours of their lives whose symptoms persist uncontrolled or unendurable despite the best efforts of experts in symptom control. Where in these circumstances does the doctors' duty lie and how should he (or she) conduct himself professionally?

In moral theory the doctors' duty taken to its logical conclusion requires him to do his utmost to follow patients' wishes and relieve their symptoms even if this requires the active (properly consented and monitored) termination of a patient's life. In circumstances in which the patient specifically asks for their life to be ended and this request is sustained over a period of time and supported by the family, it can be argued that the doctor's duty of care will ultimately require him to release the patient from their life of intolerable symptoms.

It is relatively easy to understand how patients with very severe symptoms may conclude that they would prefer not to stay alive. However, there are patients who may *not* appear to be in severe physical distress but who may nonetheless conclude that this life for them is not worth living. There are many independent-minded people who have lived active fulfilling lives, taking responsibility at every turn for their decisions, their families, and their working responsibilities. At the end of such fruitful lives these are the people who have a horror of being so ill that they are dependent on others for their care. For some people this situation is as intolerable as suffering from severe physical symptoms. How should a responsible doctor respond to a request from such a patient to help them terminate their own lives, which to them appear worthless? Equally importantly (and this a thread running through the whole of our inquiry) how can this personal and individual tragedy be reconciled with the needs of public policy?

Some doctors argue that intensive emotional and spiritual support can help the patient achieve new previously undiscovered personal horizons even at this late stage of life. They feel that the desperation which underlies the request to hasten death in those without intractable physical symptoms can be ameliorated by reducing emotional isolation, hopelessness, and fear. With intensive help patients may develop a quality of life that they see as rewarding enough to continue until death comes naturally; but they may not. It is necessary for doctors to beware of imposing their own values on their patients, assuming that these values are shared. What seems important in all these complex issues is the fact that doctors do frequently have to make value judgements.

One of the judgements that doctors quite frequently make is that a treatment which may be available is nonetheless 'futile'. Futility implies pointlessness. Either the treatment will not work, or it will result in harm, very poor quality of life, or excessive impact on family and professional carers.[4] Treatment is not obligatory when it offers no prospect of benefit to the patient. There are several classes of patients for whom there is no hope that treatment will be effective. Obviously patients who are dead cannot benefit from further treatment. The diagnosis of death is not necessarily clear, however, when considering a patient maintained on a life support machine while the criteria for determining brain death are being properly established.

Secondly, treatment is inappropriate for patients whose death is imminent or who are irreversibly dying. When it can be determined (largely as a result of medical/nursing judgement) that a patient's death is imminent and that a patient is irreversibly dying, there is no medical indication for starting or continuing treatment with curative intent. Optimal care does not mean maximal treatment and prolonging life is not the same as prolonging dying. Indeed, as others have argued cogently in recent times, the human values most appreciated by patients who are at the end of their life need to be reasserted over the technological possibilities of temporary prolongation of life.[5]

In our view, the concept of futility or pointless treatment needs to be carefully re-evaluated, especially in the modern hospital setting. That treatments can be given does not necessarily entail that they should be given. Where the likelihood of benefit is really infinitesimally small and there are side-effects and potential dangers of treatment (such as fourth line chemotherapy in advanced cancers) then a frank discussion should be held with the patient. It is very likely that the patient would choose to die relatively comfortably (and often somewhat later!) of their disease rather than dying of the unpleasant side-effects and complications of futile treatment. Such decisions, however, depend on the courage of both doctor and patient to face the true alternatives. Often doctors make the judgement that they will not even offer this last resort of treatment and will save the patient the anguish of this decision. Others will question this paternalistic approach, stressing the autonomy of the patient and their right to decide these matters for themselves. But we have argued that paternalism is not always bad. It may be the dying patient's chief source of comfort when he is too ill and tired to face making his own decisions.

Much of the 'heroic' treatment carried out for elderly patients in Western countries at the end of life could well be classified as futile, as is demonstrated by the well publicized fact that a very large proportion of an American patient's insurance costs are expended in the last two weeks of life. Clearly no long-term benefit was gained.

Futility therefore needs a recognized place in medical decision-making, and already forms one consideration in the consultation process before decisions on whether a 'Not for resuscitation' statement is appropriate for any individual patient. We believe that the principles concerning when to discontinue active intervention in favour of comfort care are a matter for society and merit discussion and an informed consensus view. If treatment is futile then life itself may be futile if the quality of life for that patient does not warrant their struggle to continue it. This is where patients may seek medical help to escape a life which to them is intolerable.

Where does the doctor's own personal conscience stand in all these matters? As mentioned earlier, doctors frequently say something like: 'my training forbids me to consider assisting a patient to commit suicide' or more certainly 'forbids me to terminate that patient's life'. 'It is against all my training which has placed patient care at the very heart of my work.' However, training in medicine evolves in response to society as time goes by and what were appropriate attitudes to patients in the last few centuries are no longer acceptable in modern practice. For example, we no longer conceal true diagnoses from patients. Certain basic tenets remain fundamental although the emphasis placed on them has changed over the years. Doctors remain dedicated to the principles of caring and avoiding harm. They seek to promote at all times the welfare and 'best interest of their patients'.

But the interpretation of 'best interest' has evolved and now takes into account at a much more fundamental level the notion of the patient as a person with a right to decide on important matters concerning his own health. We think it is time to re-examine the assertion by doctors that caring for patients in such a way as to end their life runs counter to 'all their training'. The current medical syllabus, after all, places 'patient centeredness' at the pinnacle of the aims of medical training. Patient ideas, concerns, and expectations (known in medical jargon as ICE) form an important part of history-taking, and doctors in training are taught to consult and discuss management with patients at every stage.

Young doctors recently trained and those currently under training have therefore learnt to place patient autonomy at the heart of medical practice. This generation of medical practitioners will probably find advance decisions and even a request for assisted suicide much more acceptable as part of professional practice. Medical training in itself is therefore, in our view, not a fundamental reason for the refusal of the medical profession to embrace assisted dying or euthanasia in appropriate circumstances if legislation can be effectively drafted and compassionately embraced.

At the same time, respect for the doctor's autonomy demands that doctors should have the right, if conscience dictates, to decline involvement in euthanasia or assisted suicide, in the same way as conscientious objection to participation in abortion has been respected. Nevertheless, their duty will be to refer interested patients to colleagues who can talk through these options in a balanced way, as any guidelines will require. The doctor's claim to moral conscience should not outweigh his duty of care to the patient. The doctor's right to exercise his or her conscience should not 'trump' the legitimate claim of the patient to care within the law. It will become the patient's right to get information and a referral for assisted dying once this is legal. The rather small numbers of patients ever in fact likely to request assistance with suicide will not require the participation of large numbers of doctors and may in our view be best practised by qualified 'specialists' in this practice.

In addition there is every good reason why geriatric medicine and palliative care training should form an important part of the medical curriculum. We are witnessing the expansion of an ageing population with attendant long-term problems of disability and chronic illness. Expertise in managing the last years and months of long life will be invaluable to most doctors and just as palliative care increases in its practice and importance, so also could the development of skills and decision-making guidelines for assisted dying and euthanasia, if this is what society demands.

# 9 Four Methods of Easing Death and their Effect on Doctors

The subject of dying and death is largely avoided as a topic of conversation in Britain today. This means that many people have little opportunity to express their personal views and to make choices about where and how they wish to end their days. One of the suggestions underpinning consultation on the new 'National Initiative on End of Life Care' proposed by Professor Mike Richards (National Director of Cancer Care)[1] as well as 'Advance Care Planning in Primary Care'[2] is that doctors should open the discussions about these choices much earlier in a patient's course of illness. This will enable the patient to plan more effectively and more personally for their last days.

Even in a medical setting doctors with their patients tend to avoid direct discussion of impending death. Doctors prefer to avoid distressing their patients with this stark reality and patients, understandably, often seek to defer conversations about death even when it is imminent. In oncology, for example, there may develop an element of collusion between patient and doctor with false optimism about the likelihood of recovery.[3] Many patients when they fear that their prognosis is rather poor do not ask for precise information and do not hear it if it is provided by the doctor. This topic is, however, important because patients' ideas about their prognosis affect the choices they make about their treatment and end of life care. Families who do not understand the likely course of events can misread the situation and later regret that they were not more present or more supportive at the critical time.

Not only do we need greater clarity in discussions about death but as a community we also need a wider selection of options. These options largely embrace where and under whose care we die, but also may include the timing of our own deaths.

Samples of public opinion in Britain and abroad have registered a voice for change and an indication that the public may wish to lead the medical professionals in embracing some form of assistance with the end of life. A recent British social attitude survey published in January 2007 seemed to show that 80 per cent of a large representative sample of the British public want a change in the law. Similarly, 85 per cent of a sample of 1,386 members of the Dutch general public, where euthanasia is practised, registered acceptance of active ending of life at the request of the terminally ill cancer patient. Interestingly, the same question posed to Dutch physicians gained only 64 per cent support.[4]

Palliative care is generally agreed to be the desirable standard of care for the dying when patients determine that the burdens of treatment aimed at prolonging life outweigh the benefits. Care for living reverts to care for dying, with the emphasis on symptom control, comfort, and dignity. But there remain some patients for whom intolerable suffering persists. What options currently exist within the law for offering succour to these few but worrying cases?

In the face of ethical and legal controversy about the acceptability of physician-assisted suicide and voluntary active euthanasia, the voluntary stopping of eating and drinking by the patient, perhaps combined with terminal sedation, have been proposed as ethically superior responses of last resort that do not require changes in professional standards or the law.

This theoretically humane and effective escape from the legal dilemma, apparently already in practice abroad, involves the voluntary cessation on the part of the patient of both food and drink with a view to hastening their own death. Some fortunate patients have embarked on this process with the agreed cooperation of their medical team in controlling any discomfort of hunger and thirst by simple measures, medication, or palliative sedation where necessary.

We should like to examine this proposal for what we may call 'self-denial of food and fluid' in greater detail. This course of action entails a decision on the part of an individual who is otherwise capable of taking nourishment to voluntarily deny themselves food and fluid in the full knowledge that this decision will inevitably lead to death. Depending on the patient's general state of health this process may take from a few days to a few weeks. Initially the patient may variably suffer some thirst and hunger but many severely ill patients have lost their appetite and are relieved not to feel they must eat. The principal symptom of thirst is the discomfort of a dry mouth and good mouth care is very effective at relieving this problem.

Physicians stress the fundamental role of fluids in maintaining life. The discontinuation of food alone, while continuing to take water, will not lead to the ending of life for many weeks, if not months, depending on the state of nutrition of the individual. Discontinuation of fluid intake together with abstinence from food is more rapidly fatal but even this process can be lengthy. Senior experienced specialists in palliative care have observed that even determined patients may become disheartened and give up the attempt when they find that a week or two after starting the process they are still alive.

On the other hand, in some circumstances a frail, elderly, ill, and determined patient, whose nursing and symptomatic comfort is assured, may bring about their own death within a few days by taking the decision to stop eating and drinking and carrying this through. Several individual cases are reported where patients have successfully prepared themselves and their family and are at peace with the world. After stopping all intake these patients have lasted between three and fifteen days.[5]

The discontinuation of hydration in patients dying naturally has caused a great deal of disagreement among palliative care specialists. Some believe that water is the very elixir of life and that to deprive a patient of intravenous fluids if they cannot on their own take even sips of fluid is cruel. Through the ages the giving of food and drink has been symbolic of care and compassion and in modern medicine this translates to intravenous, naso-gastric or direct gastric feeding. Nurses in particular may find the withholding of fluids directly in conflict with professional instincts.

Others have observed that giving a thirsty patient intravenous fluid does not in fact relieve their thirst, but may aggravate the accumulation of fluid peripherally as ascites (swollen abdomen), swollen limbs, and pulmonary oedema (excess fluid compressing the lungs). In medical terms it is very common in the dying that central dehydration and peripheral oedema exist together. There have also been observations by nurses and physicians alike that dehydration can indeed increase comfort, perhaps by relieving pressure on diseased organs.[6] Towards the end of life it appears that an electrolyte balance is created naturally to cope with the changing situation.

Most patients who stop taking food and fluids do not in fact complain of thirst, and keeping the mouth moist with sips of fluid or ice-cubes and dry lips comfortable with cream is much more effective than an intravenous drip at controlling the sensation of thirst.

Because of the resolve and determination needed to discontinue eating and drinking there can be no doubt as to the voluntary nature of this decision on the patient's part. Both ethically and legally the right of an individual to refuse treatment, including food and water, is well established (see Bland[7]) and the voluntary cessation of 'natural' eating and drinking can be seen as an extension of that right.[8] This decision also protects patient privacy and independence even as far as, in theory, not requiring the participation of a doctor at all (not in our view an advisable approach). Many patients who fear prolonged suffering and lack of choice find this possibility reassuring because it does not require 'permission' from the healthcare team. Ideally clinicians participate in the initial evaluation and then palliate symptoms throughout the course. This process need not compromise public confidence in the medical profession because it does not require the doctor to assume any new role or responsibility beyond their normal role as healer, caregiver, and counsellor.

A number of disadvantages are nonetheless evident. This may be a lengthy process placing intolerable anguish on the family and professional carers. It is very hard to watch a loved one die slowly of starvation and dehydration. It is difficult for carers to know whether to offer fluids, thereby increasing comfort but undermining the patient's avowed intent. If fluids are not offered, on the other hand, this may be read as coercion to proceed with the process. If doctors are not involved, for example, when a patient undertakes this process unsupervised at home, proper informed decision-making may be lacking, cases of treatable depression may be missed, and symptom control may be inadequate. Patients are likely to lose mental clarity as this process proceeds and if proper advanced instructions have not been given doubt may be raised about the continued voluntary nature of the process. On the point of death some families tend to panic and bring the dying patient to the emergency department. This is a very unsatisfactory outcome for all concerned.

On the other hand, in the hospital or hospice setting severe symptoms can be more readily and confidently controlled during the dying process. A small number of patients will embark on this self-denial process in order, as they see it, to escape from symptoms which even modern palliative medicine is unable to control. Estimates of the frequency of refractory symptoms vary between 16 per cent of hospice patients[9] and 50 per cent of hospital patients.[10] Symptoms may be intractable either because treatment is ineffective or the treatment itself is intolerable.

In such circumstances of distress these patients may request some sedation to at least 'take the edge off' the awareness of their predicament. The use of 'terminal sedation' to control the intense discomfort of dying patients appears to have become an established practice in some centres of palliative care. Fainsinger and colleagues[11] for example described the use of sedation during the last week of life in four hospice settings in Israel, Cape Town, Durban, and Madrid. The length of time for which sedation was required was consistent between the centres (1-6 days), as was the dosage used (usually Midazolam). More than 90 per cent of patients needed standard medication for symptoms such as pain, dyspnoea, nausea, and vomiting. The intention to bring in sedation varied from 15 to 36 per cent of cases, the commonest indication for sedation being agitated confusion (delirium). The term 'terminal sedation' is in fact poorly defined. The intention of this sedation varies from controlled carefully measured sedation with the aim of just relieving a patient's distress, to heavy sedation producing drug-induced coma which persists until the patient dies of their disease. Such lack of precision makes an analysis of the place of sedation in end of life care difficult to clarify. A further review of palliative sedation in Spain[12] is difficult to interpret because of this variation in intention. Some doctors intentionally sedated patients to coma levels before death, while others simply used light sedation to relieve distress.

An important issue in the debate about terminal sedation is the extent to which it differs from euthanasia. Some argue that, because terminal sedation is aimed at alleviating the symptoms of anxiety and emotional distress, it is quite distinct from euthanasia. The patient dies of their underlying fatal disease in relatively greater comfort. Others, however, regard this as a specious distinction, because the intention of true terminal sedation is not to allow the patient to recover consciousness before death supervenes. The claim of the intention of double effect would therefore not seem to apply. The intention is single, that the patient should die under sedation. In our view there are two distinct forms of sedation which need to regarded separately.

In practice in the UK the use of appropriate sedation at the end of life is much more accurately described as 'palliative sedation' than 'terminal sedation' and would seem to clearly intend symptom control as distinct from euthanasia (which is currently of course illegal). The intention is careful escalation of sedation, usually using Midazolam (not morphine), to a level which just controls mental or physical anguish as demonstrated by facial expression or bodily restlessness.

Experienced doctors and nursing staff are very clear that it is possible to tell when an unconscious patient is suffering. When patients are unrousable their facial expression nonetheless reflects their level of both physical and emotional distress. Frowning with deep vertical creasing is a manifestation of marked distress as well as facial grimacing. These signs can be seen in the unconscious patient, and are non-verbal signs of distress. When adequate analgesia is given, starting at a low dose and working carefully upwards, the facial expression clears. If the patient looks at peace then one can be confident that they are not conscious of distress. Emotional turmoil is also manifest both facially and physically throughout the body, with evidence of agitation and restlessness.

The question arises as to how best to help unconscious but restless patients if they are beyond the reach of the reassurance of the presence of loved ones or the calming effects of touch, massage, music, or for some the reading of religious texts. With experienced clinical expertise it is possible to deepen unconsciousness to a level that is more comfortable for the patient. This is now usually achieved with subcutaneous Midazolam titrated (evaluated) against the patient's response, starting with a low dose and working up to what appears necessary for the patient to be at peace.

It is a question much discussed as to whether this kind of use of opioids or sedative drugs is hastening death. A recent report in the journal *Lancet Oncology* comprehensively reviewed the evidence on this point.[13] The authors analysed seventeen studies which examined the use of opioids at the end of life and a further seventeen studies that addressed the use of sedatives in the care of cancer patients in the final stages of life. They also viewed the results from an ethical perspective to establish whether the doctrine of double effect had been required to justify the drugs and doses used. They concluded that patients are more likely to receive higher doses of both opioids and sedatives as they get closer to death. However they found *no* evidence that initiation of treatment or increases in doses were associated with precipitation of death. They concluded that the doctrine of double effect was not essential for the justification of these drugs.

In a further inquiry into the practice of sedation at their own institution these authors then reviewed the case notes of 237 consecutive cases who died in their specialist palliative care unit.[14] Survival after admission was compared between groups of patients receiving no sedation, sedation for seven days, or a commencement of sedation in the last forty-eight hours of life. Sedation was given to 48 per cent of patients. Sedative use and dose increased in the last hours of life but were not associated with shortened survival overall. The number of days between admission and death proved to be the same whether sedation was used or not.

In our view it is high time this misapprehension was laid to rest. The fear that death is being hastened by what is in fact correct use and dose of these medications has led unnecessarily to a fear on the part of doctors of accusations of malpractice. The result appears to be that patients in extremis may be being denied effective symptom control. (Morphine kills the pain, not the patient.)[15]

In summary, the concept of self-denial of food and fluids combined with appropriate sedation for symptom management appears to offer a legitimate means for patients to end their lives with the cooperation of the healthcare team. Voluntarily stopping eating and drinking combined with palliative sedation allows doctors to remain responsive to a wide range of patient suffering.

## Four Methods of Easing Death

Some however claim that this process could also be interpreted as the doctor aiding and abetting suicide, in that the patient's intention is clear and the administration of sedation could be regarded as preventing the patient changing their mind about pursuing suicide.

Whatever the process adopted, safeguards are required for any medical action that may hasten death, including determining that palliative care is being ineffective, obtaining informed consent, ensuring diagnostic and prognostic clarity, obtaining an independent second opinion, implementing reporting and monitoring processes and a reflective pause. (All of these safeguards were included in Lord Joffe's Bill in the UK.)

In our view, however, the simple expedient of self-denial of food and fluids does not seem to supply an answer for many patients who seek to end their lives. The discomfort involved in starvation and dehydration may be manageable, but the sheer length of the dying process is frequently inhumane. This seems to us essentially a legitimate way to avoid the current unintentionally inhumane legal framework regulating assisted dying (Suicide Act 1961, the Homicide Act 1957).

Physician-assisted suicide, on the other hand, places control of the timing of death firmly in the patient's hands. The doctor, or perhaps a specialized service similar to that in Switzerland, provides the means, usually a prescription of a large dose of barbiturates by which a patient can end his or her life. Although the doctor is morally responsible for this assistance, patients have to carry out the final act themselves. Many doctors are much more willing to contemplate this kind of process than euthanasia because there is at least a shared responsibility and a little more distance between the doctor's role and the patient's death.

Assisted dying has several advantages. For some patients access to a lethal dose of medication may give them the confidence and reassurance to go on living, knowing they can escape if and when they choose. This possibility of escape is extremely important to many people. Evidence from the Death with Dignity programme in Oregon demonstrates that only about half of those patients who sought the wherewithal to take their lives actually needed this in the end.[16]

Typically patients continue their lives, accepting or declining active treatment until such time as the burden of life outweighs its pleasures. The most obvious advantage of assisted dying over self-denial of food and water is the predictable time-scale and the dignity and control which remain within the patient's power. Patients take their dose at a moment of their choosing, when it is still within their physical power to do so. Because patients need to administer the medication themselves their action is most likely to be voluntary.

One serious drawback immediately appears. Patients who suffer from conditions making it difficult for them to swallow or control other important voluntary movements may have the clarity of mind to make the decision to take a lethal dose but someone suffering from, for example, motor neurone disease, as did Mrs Diane Pretty, would lack the ability actually to carry out her necessary part in the procedure. (The case of Mrs Pretty was discussed in detail in Chapter 1.) It would be sadly paradoxical if the law were changed, at least in part because of the widespread publicity of Diane Pretty's case and the sympathy it evoked, but it were changed in such a way that it would not have benefited her, and other sufferers from motor neurone disease. Yet if a Bill permitting assisted suicide were proposed, which had an exemption only for those suffering from motor neurone disease, who alone might be directly caused to die,

**113**

then at once the full force of the slippery slope argument would be brought to bear to prevent its passage. If one exemption, why not others? The inevitability of further extension into euthanasia would be argued.

Assisted suicide also has some practical disadvantages. First, of course, as we have said, many doctors and nurses find the idea repugnant and, although this may change over time, not all patients would find their own doctor sympathetic and would need to be referred on. Secondly, self-administration of drugs can misfire. The patient may take the wrong dose or vomit after taking the medication. They may not be thinking clearly at that time and may in fact be acting under duress if the process is not properly supervised and monitored. Self-medication is not always effective and a family may be faced with a patient who is vomiting, confused, or comatose but not dying. Patients brought to the emergency department are likely to be given unwanted life-prolonging treatment. For this reason doctors in the Netherlands have made it their practice to be on hand to administer euthanasia if assisted suicide should fail. This backup would not of course be available in Britain if new legislation were to be restricted to assisted suicide only.

With voluntary active euthanasia, the doctor, or a specially trained team, not only provides the means but is the final actor by administering a fatal injection at the patient's request. As practised in the Netherlands, there is a lengthy process of discussion and preparation. Once all the conditions of the policy have been satisfied the patient is sedated to unconsciousness and then given a lethal injection of a muscle-paralysing agent like curare. For patients who are determined to die because their suffering is intolerable, euthanasia has the advantage of being quick and effective. Patients do not need to be able to swallow or have manual dexterity and this may be of great benefit to the small numbers of patients with neurological disorders who seek this way out. Because doctors are directly involved with the procedure it is easier to ensure that all the guidelines have been followed, that the patient's decision is consistent and truly voluntary, that the diagnosis and prognosis are correctly established, that all other palliative options have been properly explored, and that no duress is evident. The Netherlands is the only country so far where voluntary active euthanasia (and physician-assisted suicide) are openly practised, regulated, and studied. Yet only approximately 2 per cent of all deaths result from euthanasia and 0.2–0.4 per cent of deaths result from physician-assisted suicide. The numbers involved are not great but are nonetheless important for the intensity of suffering which is alleviated.

Of concern is the report that, in 0.7–0.8 per cent of deaths, active euthanasia in Holland was performed on patients who had lost the capacity to consent, raising concerns as to whether guidelines restricting euthanasia to competent patients and those with valid advanced directives can be enforced in practice.[17] More recent Dutch reports (2007) have been reassuring on this point.[18] First, the incidence of euthanasia without patient consent did not increase between 2001 and 2005. Secondly, in the majority of these cases doctors were responding to the previously expressed wishes of the patient with the agreement of the family and/or a second physician. But, as we have already noticed, statistics on what is an illegal practice are unlikely to be very reliable.

Doctors in the Netherlands, where terminal care is largely managed by the family doctor at home, have stressed the importance for them of a long association with a patient who ultimately requests help to die. In the UK where palliative care may be conducted by a

GP group practice but is increasingly the realm of specialist hospice teams, a long acquaintance with a given patient is quite unusual.

Hospice teams have at least one major hesitation in being involved with assisted dying or euthanasia. The hospice movement has won an honoured place in most communities and has a powerful reputation for tireless care and support for dying patients and their families. In addition hospice staff are frequently regarded with greater respect and trust than any professional the patient will so far have encountered in the management of his medical problems. Patients know that the palliative care team is completely committed to their welfare in a way which other staff have had more difficulty in delivering.

Yet Hospice Care receives only 25-30 per cent of its revenue from the government. The bulk of the financial support of each local hospice comes from the voluntary support of the local community. Hospice administrators are seriously concerned that any association of hospices with assisted suicide or euthanasia will confuse the public and diminish the community's enthusiastic support, to the detriment of the existing excellent services.

So far our contemplation of issues at the end of life has concentrated on the patient and the family. But what of the health professionals involved? What toll, if any, do these procedures take on the staff called upon to be involved? How do doctors themselves feel if they have been instrumental in a patient's death either through euthanasia or physician-assisted suicide?

Several studies have addressed this question in different countries. Since euthanasia has been tolerated and practised in the Netherlands for many decades this country provides the majority of evidence of the practice of euthanasia. Haverkate and colleagues[19] reported on 'the emotional impact on physicians of hastening the death of a patient' in the Netherlands in 2001. At that time both euthanasia and assisted suicide were still criminal offences, but the penal code had been amended to exempt doctors from criminal liability if they reported their actions and showed that they had satisfied the requirements for prudent practice. A random sample of 405 doctors was interviewed between 1995 and 1996. The data on the feelings of the physicians after perceived hastening of the death of a patient were available for three categories: cases of euthanasia, assisted suicide, and cases of ending life without an explicit request from the patient. In approximately half of all cases physicians reported that they had feelings of comfort afterwards, while feelings of discomfort were reported by slightly less than half. The greater the degree of suffering on the part of the patient, the more likely was a feeling of comfort for the physician later. Doctors who had previously performed euthanasia reported that their most recent case of euthanasia had been just as difficult as earlier cases. It seemed that the number of cases of euthanasia or assisted suicide performed by a physician made little difference to the strength of the reported emotional impact. Repeated performance did not appear to 'numb the emotions' or render this emotionally laden type of medical decision part of 'normal' medical practice. The overwhelming majority of physicians stated that they would be willing to perform euthanasia or assisted suicide again in similar circumstances. In 85 per cent of cases, the physician thought that the quality of dying had been improved considerably by euthanasia and in 67 per cent of cases the physician thought that the quality of dying had been improved considerably by assisted suicide.

Among the 159 physicians who had performed euthanasia 43 per cent later sought support in coping. Most often support was found privately among friends, family, and colleagues. Overall, the Dutch experience reported in 2001 showed that granting the ultimate wish of a competent patient may give many physicians a feeling of having contributed positively to the quality of patient care and the dying process. In Holland some doctors commented after helping their patient to die that this completed their clinical duty, saying: 'It is the last thing I can do for my patient'.[20]

A few years later Obstein *et al.* questioned thirty Dutch family physicians in northern Holland who had been known to participate in the programme of euthanasia.[21] The thirty physicians interviewed had conducted euthanasia on average once every 2.8 years. All those interviewed stated that all of their experiences of euthanasia had been positive to some degree and that if they had not felt positive about a case they would not have been involved. Many stressed the importance of being able to help a patient in the patient's time of greatest suffering. None had regrets about the cases of euthanasia they had performed. Many of the physicians described a 'conflict' between heart and mind. The heart resisted taking a life, as it felt an unnatural act to any human being, especially to a physician. The mind however overpowered the heart in acknowledging that, by conducting euthanasia, the physician is acting in a humane manner towards the patient. The majority of these doctors' patients had actually died naturally due to illness and euthanasia made up a very small proportion of deaths in their medical practice. The majority of their patients usually did not know that they had conducted euthanasia during their career. However, the patients who did know, or who asked about euthanasia, were glad to learn that their physician was receptive to the idea.

Physicians commented that euthanasia caused them to think about life and death more frequently, causing them to wonder more deeply about the meaning of life and the importance of living life to its greatest potential. Most of these doctors also developed a support system, usually including family members, friends, and colleagues. Because each physician spent weeks or months debating whether euthanasia would be appropriate for their individual suffering patient, they did wonder whether their attention to this process and their focus on the patient resulted in less attention paid to their own family and friends. They described the act of euthanasia as more of a rigorous process than an isolated procedure. All stated that they were confident that their duty as doctors was upheld. This study reports many specific comments from doctors of which this is typical: 'all the cases are positive for me ... The problem could not be solved another way.'

In the United States, where these procedures remain either illegal or only recently legalized, doctors also found the experience to be profound and time-consuming. Emmanuel and colleagues analysed the practice of euthanasia and physician assisted suicide in the United States.[22] During this study in-depth interviews were conducted with a total of 355 oncologists, 38 of whom had carried out either euthanasia or physician-assisted suicide. In about a quarter of the cases of potential physician-assisted suicide, the patients never actually used the medication for suicide and in a further 15 per cent of these cases the attempted suicide failed.

The majority of US oncologists found comfort in knowing that they had 'helped the patient end his or her life the way the patient wished'. A quarter of oncologists, however, regretted performing euthanasia or physician-assisted suicide. While some of these oncologists feared prosecution as a result of their action, it is clear from the interviews that regrets resulted from other concerns. Some doctors expressed worries about 'playing God a little bit too much' and conveyed a sense that ending a patient's life made physicians feel 'conflicted, at odds with myself and my role'. A third of oncologists felt that the emotional burden associated with these decisions affected the way they practised medicine. Some stated that it made them listen to their patients with more insight and sympathy. Others, however, found that the emotional burden had an adverse effect. For some it made them avoid situations in the future that might lead to another request for euthanasia or physician-assisted suicide.

It is worth stressing that this review was conducted at a time when neither euthanasia nor physician-assisted suicide was legal in any part of the United States. As a result, the carefully prepared and well accepted safeguards in use in Holland and now in Oregon were not a formal part of these end of life procedures. The procedures used did not necessarily ensure that these requests were initiated by the patient, voluntary, and well considered. The authors found it particularly disturbing that in 15 per cent of cases the patients themselves were not involved in the decision, but it was the family who wanted the patient's life ended. Because euthanasia and physician-assisted suicide were illegal when the interviews were conducted, it is understandable that US physicians were unwilling to consult a colleague about a request and thus a second opinion was less often sought than would be required in any regulated system. One potential important problem arose. The authors found that in 15 per cent of physician-assisted suicide attempts the patient failed to die. Such failures may occur because physicians do not know what medications to prescribe to end patients' lives or because patients do not take the life-ending medication appropriately. In the Netherlands the ethos is that physicians should be within close proximity and be willing to perform euthanasia if the patient's attempted suicide fails. This approach is unlikely to work in the

United Kingdom. First, it appears that if any life-ending intervention were to be legalized, it would be to permit physician-assisted suicide only. Thus euthanasia to remedy a failed suicide case is likely to remain illegal. Further it has emerged that physicians who are willing to perform physician-assisted suicide are often unwilling to perform euthanasia. These doctors find such a role too active. Thus legalizing physician-assisted suicide, but not euthanasia, could create serious difficulties in addressing the failed suicide attempt.

In summary the majority of these US oncologists would perform euthanasia and assisted suicide again in a similar case and received comfort from having helped a patient. Nevertheless a significant minority of oncologists experienced substantial problems from their actions. In almost a quarter of cases physicians regretted performing euthanasia or assisted suicide after the incident and in almost one in six cases physicians experienced emotional distress.

Of concern was the sense of isolation that doctors felt from their colleagues and their medical institutions. Even in Oregon, where physician-assisted suicide is now legally permitted, under clearly specified circumstances, the controversy surrounding the process still made physicians reluctant to share this profound experience with colleagues. It appears that, because palliative care is much less well developed in the United States, there is not yet the readiness to sit down and explore the practice and the emotional aspects of such requests. Frequently the underlying suffering that is motivating the request for euthanasia (undertreated symptoms, a family crisis, a spiritual crisis, or clinical depression) can be responded to directly, alleviating the need for an assisted death.[23] Educational efforts are needed to prepare physicians to explore the meaning of such requests, to exclude depression as the motivation and to ensure the adequacy of palliative care.[24]

## Four Methods of Easing Death

Of moral interest is the observation that highly ethical and humane physicians have been known to assist their colleagues and their loved ones to have a more merciful death in contrast to their normal practice with the majority of their patients. 'That physicians and nurses would request euthanasia for their colleagues or would assist their loved ones to have a more merciful death...says something about the moral nature of the act.'[25] The fact that experienced doctors (who after all understand thoroughly what dying entails) have been known to set aside their fear of legal repercussions in order to smooth the dying path for friends and loved ones implies that this assistance is inherently a moral and loving act.[26]

It is difficult to assess to what degree the doctors' distress would be improved by bringing these end of life practices into the open and into the mainstream of accepted medical practice. Alternatively, it has been suggested that an end of life service staffed by technicians, properly trained and supported by doctors, nurses, pharmacologists, and psychologists would go a long way to obviating these difficulties. This might be one solution to allow for a predictable response for the few whose suffering becomes intolerable in spite of optimal palliative care. On the other hand, doctors in Holland were clear that, if requested to carry out euthanasia, they felt much more comfortable helping a patient who had been known to them a long time.[27] It is in our view preferable that assisted dying, if legalized, should remain under medical supervision, perhaps in the hands of specialist physicians who favour this approach and can offer continuity of care and a final act of friendship.

So, from a medical standpoint, what do we conclude is the path forward to assist those suffering severely at the end of their lives? In our view, although strong arguments exist for the role of voluntary euthanasia in selected cases, society may not be yet ready to embrace these. Although assisted suicide and euthanasia are morally equivalent, nonetheless for pragmatic reasons we favour confining legal change in the foreseeable future to assisted suicide.

A wise policy may be to legislate to permit assisted suicide in a carefully considered manner, developing a strategy to ensure adherence to safe guidelines and with diligent monitoring to assess the effect of such a policy on public opinion, attitudes to the vulnerable, prevention of inappropriate duress, and attitudes to euthanasia itself. We are however seriously concerned that, because assisted suicide is not infallible and things can go wrong, the doctor agreeing to help his patient to die should take some responsibility for that failure and be prepared to ensure the patient's continuing welfare.

We believe that debate in this area should no longer be dominated by a minority of critical, often faith-led voices who may be doctors themselves, but should be responsive to the views of the majority of the community. Those who disagree have every right to voice their disapproval and not to participate but they should not impose their convictions on the quiet majority.

Whichever choice society makes to address the symptoms of the small numbers of patients whose suffering is irremediable at the end of life, an explicit public policy about which of these practices are permissible would reassure the many patients in fear of their future and their death.

# 10 Looking Further Ahead

A t the end of the last chapter we cautiously recommended that new legislation be introduced that would permit assisted suicide for those competent patients who asked for it, subject to stringent safeguards. However in the same chapter we recognized that both the moral attitudes of society and the education of doctors are far from static and immutable. They change over time. In this chapter we consider some ways in which attitudes towards death may change, indeed have already changed; and we suggest that this may have consequences for the law, consequences that will not be disastrous, as some people fear, but on the contrary may lead to a more civilized and compassionate society.

In opposing Lord Joffe's Bill on assisted dying, Lord Habgood, former archbishop of York, employed a version of the slippery slope argument (see Chapter 7 above) less speculative than some others. He predicted that if there were any relaxation in the law prohibiting assisted death, whether assisted suicide or euthanasia, society would become accustomed to the idea, and this would lead to a cultural change: a change in the way we look at ourselves and others. It would be a change of values; but, more than that, it would involve a conceptual shift, a new way of perceiving what it is to be a human being.[1] In principle, we accept this argument; but we do not believe that it provides a reason that the law should not be changed. For there are at least two conceptual changes that have already taken place, and society cannot go back. They form part of the atmosphere at the top of the slope where we stand, rather than lurking as a quagmire to be dreaded at the bottom. We will try to explain the nature of these changes, without either praising or deploring them, for they are simply matters of history, part of the way we live now.

The first change is social, and we have frequently remarked on it already. We hardly need reminding that people live much longer than they used to. It is true that there are still killer diseases such as AIDS; and there are parts of the world where life expectancy is less than half what it is in the West. We are always at risk of a lethal pandemic that will kill millions, besides those who die of starvation, in natural disasters, or in war. Nevertheless, these deaths, which shock us, do so in part because they occur in a world where hygiene has found ways to protect us against many diseases, and medicine and surgery have found cures for others. In February 2006 the British Government Actuary Department published their calculation that in seventy years time 1.2 million Britons will live to be 100, and many thousands will reach the age of 110.

Increased longevity has two somewhat conflicting consequences. The first is that we may come to think that death, being something that can be almost indefinitely fended off, ought necessarily to be fended off; it is an avoidable disaster. But, secondly, we no longer have the tradition of cohesive families, within which the old play an important and useful part; where at the end of their lives they are cared for and protected by those for whom they have previously

cared and provided, and are finally seen off, ready to die, and sur-
rounded by their family. We may greatly admire those who still
thus look after their aged parents, and we may regret the change
(though we may also perhaps sentimentalize it). But we cannot fail
to acknowledge the sociological fact that a majority of the very old
now spend their last months or years in hospitals or 'care homes'
where, for many, their death is the result of a decision, not their own,
that the effort to keep them alive may properly be abandoned, and
they are deliberately allowed to die. We proclaim the belief that the
civilization of a society is measured by the care it takes of its most
vulnerable members, including the very old. Yet not only are we
frequently shocked by stories of neglect, but, more fundamentally,
we are forced to ask ourselves what all the extra years that people
live are actually worth to the people who live them. As the journalist
Mary Riddell put it, 'making people more death-proof is easy. The
hard thing is going to be working out what all that extra life is really
for.'[2] This question is most insistent when old people have reached
a condition where their consciousness is totally absorbed by pain
and distress, or where they have lapsed into dementia.

So the way things are in society has already brought about a
change in our attitudes, causing us to question openly, in a manner
previously unthinkable, the way the end of life is managed for an
increasing number of people. It is no longer enough simply to throw
up our hands in horror and cry that we cannot allow the weak to be
deprived of their right to life, or that we are heading for the horrors
of the concentration camps. Nor is it enough, however reluctantly,
to conclude with Professor Biggar that the sanctity of human life
demands the sacrifice of a few people who are suffering and forced
to continue to live for the sake of the good of the majority (see
Chapter 6). The numbers are by now too many. His argument that

'extreme cases' should not be allowed to determine policy, because they are so few will not really hold for the future, whether we are thinking of patients in PVS (who are not in fact suffering) or of those who truly suffer.

There has been another and more philosophical change as well, more concerned with our background presuppositions about human nature than about social circumstances. Gradually, since Darwin, we have become accustomed to placing human beings among the other animals, and all animals among the rest of nature. Human life remains, in the eyes of most of us, a uniquely important form of life. The human brain has features to be found in no other animal. We value human life above all else, because it is among other human beings that we have our traceable genetic origins, our morality, our loyalties, our loves, and our hopes for the future. We are social animals and the society of which we are part is made up of our own species. But human life is nevertheless different only in its degree of complexity from other forms. All living things are natural organisms, and just as we cannot separate the body from the soul of plants and animals, their outer from their inner life, so we cannot any longer, most of us, make such a separation in human beings.

Think, for example, of our understanding of the habits of birds We are still relatively ignorant of their brain-functions, how much they can learn, how much they can improvise (as in the construction of nests out of new materials), and how much is 'instinctive', built into their genetic inheritance. Our situation is not much different if we contemplate our own species. And when we speak of genes or of the adaptations and connexions within the brain, we are speaking of the body, that aspect of the physiology of the organism that gives rise to experience. We are not speaking of something added on, inserted from the outside and therefore theoretically at least capable of independence, the Mind or Soul.

As Peter Strawson argued in his seminal work *Individuals*, we cannot think of human persons in any way except as both corporeal objects and as subjects with states of consciousness, the very same identical individuals having both features properly ascribed to them.[3] And he concludes from this that the idea of the 'pure ego', the self that is nothing but the receptor of inner experience, is empty. The fact that we communicate with one another about our perceptions, our feelings, and our thoughts shows that language itself does not arise within a uniquely separate internal 'mind', but comes into existence in an already perceived communality of experiences, both 'inner' and 'outer'. The nature of language demands that we language-users share both the 'subjective' and the 'objective' aspects of experience. That is what it came into existence for, and why it is, to a large extent, successful in communicating.

Descartes held that man consisted of two quite separate substances, the thinking substance (*res cogitans*) and the material substance (*res extensa*). For him it was an intractable problem to account for the fact that we believe, as we do, that anything exists outside our own personal and 'private' experience, let alone that we talk to other people about it. Edmund Husserl and the German phenomenologists of the early twentieth century were the first to insist on the unity of the inner and the outer. It was a revolutionary idea. The answer to Descartes's problem of how we can be sure that the external world exists at all, except as an idea in our own mind, a dream, was simply that it was not a problem. We are ourselves part of the 'external world'. It is the only world there is. The sole difference between ourselves and stones and trees is that consciousness allows us and other animals to be aware of, as well as part of, the world. In 1939 Sartre, on coming back from Germany where he had been studying the works of Husserl, wrote in excitement: 'We are delivered from the "internal life"…since everything is finally outside, everything, even ourselves. Outside in the world among others. It is not in some hiding-place that we will find ourselves: it is on the road, in the town, in the midst of the crowd, a thing among things, a man among men.'[4]

According to Sartre, Husserl had exorcised what the British philosopher Gilbert Ryle later called the Ghost in the Machine, the 'official doctrine', he said, of dualism, derived from Descartes, but shared by 'most philosophers, psychologists and religious teachers'. This was the doctrine of mind separate from but inhabiting body.[5] Ryle, unlike most English-speaking philosophers at the time, was well acquainted with the works of the German phenomenologists (though his style was conspicuously different from theirs). He was also acquainted with the developing ideas of that most influential of twentieth-century philosophers, Ludwig Wittgenstein (himself strongly influenced, one may suspect, by Husserl, though this was never acknowledged, for he preferred to think of himself as an unlettered genius). In his later writings Wittgenstein too urged us to forget the Cartesian image of our each having something secretly within us, where our sensations, emotions, and perceptions, our consciousness of them and the words we use of them lie hidden.[6] To say of someone that he is aware of his surroundings is simply to say that, being an animal and part of the world, he is conscious of it. He is not a material body which 'has' within his mind certain 'sense-data' or 'ideas' the relation of which to the outside world is problematic. However mysterious and ill-understood consciousness may be, and whatever happens in our brains when we learn about our surroundings, there is, as Sartre put it, only one world. A human being is a 'thing among things' as well as a 'man among men'. This dismantling of dualism constituted, as has been said, a revolution in philosophy in the first half of the twentieth century.

It may, understandably, be objected that this is all highly esoteric stuff. Who heeds the disputes of philosophers? Surely the presumptions of ordinary people are never influenced by the writings of a few academics? But the words of philosophers have a way of trickling down through other discourse, that of teachers, journalists, novelists, and critics. Or perhaps philosophers themselves do no more than attempt to articulate and formalize thoughts that are already in the air, drifting about ever since the scientific revolutions of palaeontology and Darwinian gradualism.

Yet common sense and ordinary language still incline to distinguish the mental from the physical, the inner from the outer, the ghost from the machine. And one can easily enough understand why. We cannot see the changes that take place in our bodies (including, of course, our brains), when, for example, our mood changes, our resolution weakens, or our pleasure ceases. All we can do is notice what we feel, and strive to find shared words (or images or music) in which we can articulate it to ourselves or others. It is because the workings of the brain are both invisible and incomprehensible to common sense that we are inclined to think of our thoughts and feelings, the centre of our self-awareness, as made of a completely different stuff from that which other people see, our bodies, or even that which scientists can chart, the changes in our brains recorded on encephalographs, or visible on scans. And therefore we are inclined to think of the ghost as separable from the machine, with a life of its own. We may incline to think that what happens to the body is in a sense irrelevant to what happens to the real person within. Common sense finds it hard to embrace the fact that a person is one organism, whose corporeal and mental life cannot be prised apart.

Thus in giving evidence to the House of Lords Select Committee it was not wholly surprising to find the MP Mrs Curtis-Thomas speaking of the body and the spirit as 'two entirely different entities', the one remaining intact whatever the decrepitude or disintegration of the other.[7] Such extreme Cartesianism is perhaps unusual today; but it is still very much a part of the language of religion. It is hard, without faith, to believe in the unchanged endurance of the spirit, when contemplating someone in the last stages of dementia, when their whole personality has changed. Would Mrs Curtis-Thomas use the same language of her terminally sick cat? Descartes held that animals have no souls and are automata, their behaviour entirely explicable by mechanical laws, in this wholly different from human beings. If Mrs Curtis-Thomas would not use her argument to justify refusing to put down her cat when it was terminally suffering, that is, if she would assert the separability of the body from the spirit only in the case of human beings, then it seems that she must reject the Darwinian connexion between man and other animals. She must hold that our species, and it alone, was formed in the image of God, who gave it the gift of spirit or soul, along with the gift of life. In effect, then, her argument is a religious argument, asserting the sanctity of human, but only of human life.

And so, though ordinary language may still have embedded in it the relics of dualism, it is only those who are convinced of the literal truth of the religious doctrine that there exists a special relationship between man and God, the God who 'ensouls' each foetus during pregnancy, who any longer maintain a total separation of powers, if one may put it so, between the body and the soul or spirit.

This amounts to a change in culture that has to a large extent already taken place. We already tend to think of human beings in a way that is, relatively speaking, new (though we could if we liked trace it back to Aristotle, who held that man was a rational animal). The new perception of what it is to be human in no way diminishes the limitless value we attach to human beings, to the works of the human imagination, to human inventiveness and vision, including the great visions of religion.

So how does this changed perception affect the force of Lord Habgood's version of the slippery slope? It means, in reality, that there is no slope to fear, but that we have to admit and examine the new concept of mankind, the place of human beings in the natural order, and its implication for their life and death. Such an examination was hinted at in the Second Reading debate on Lord Joffe's second Bill by Baroness Richardson of Calow. Baroness Richardson is a minister in the Methodist Church, and is deeply committed to Christianity. It is worth quoting part of what she said in support of the Bill.

There is no doubt that this Bill has shocked the religious communities. It shocked us because we have had to look at ourselves in a new light. It has undermined the security that some have felt that God is in control of life and death, and that therefore our responsibility has to be simply to assist him in what is the best we can arrange; the most comfort, the deepest love, and the highest level of care. Into the hands of men and women has now been put a great responsibility over life and death, and it is no longer safe to talk about 'natural life' as though we have defined it. We do not like the thought of having the right over life and death. If we have in our hands the means by which a person can end their suffering we must ask 'What are the moral judgements we must make to withhold that?'...I hope that the debate continues in society on the value, quality and dignity of life and our responsibility for it.[8]

These are wise and significant words. If we have abandoned, or are gradually abandoning, the idea of the soul as that part of the human being that is especially God's responsibility, we have urgent questions to ask regarding our own responsibility for our own and other people's death.

First, why should we strive to keep alive those people whose body and brain together have collapsed into irreversible dysfunction? Biologically they are still alive, but what constituted the value, for them, of living has gone. They are sometimes disparagingly referred to as 'vegetables'; and their life is indeed like that of a vegetable, without self-consciousness, and only the most rudimentary awareness of pain and pleasure, or no awareness at all. The pointlessness of keeping them alive is now generally recognized for patients who are certainly in PVS, even if it must be a court of law that comes to the decision that they may be allowed to die. The judgment of the court in the case of Tony Bland is widely (though, as we have seen, not universally) agreed to have been right. But it is arguable that society, with its new concept of human life, may come openly to allow that it is futile to keep alive those who are in the last stages of dementia, who have lost the capacity to recognize the sensory input they still receive; or those who have suffered severe stroke, and who, if they continue to live, will have serious and irreparable brain damage. The most crucial, and to them inexpressibly valuable part of their body, their brain, has been ruined beyond repair. The Guidance first issued by the British Medical Association in 1999 endorses the withholding or withdrawal of tube-delivered food and water not only from patients in PVS but also from other non-terminally ill patients such as those with severe dementia or serious stroke.[9] We argued in Chapter 9 that doctors already have to make life or death decisions about when further treatment, including tube-feeding and hydration, would be 'futile', and that the concept of futility should be taken seriously as a guide to medical conduct. The BMA guidelines presumably rely on this concept of futility.

In part following other writers, such as Nigel Biggar and Ronald Dworkin, we may distinguish between biological and (auto)biographical life. Autobiographical life can be thought of as a story, coherently connected, one part with another, the central character of which is someone who recognizes himself as a unique individual who 'has' or possesses his own experiences, in the present, and at least partially in the past. Ronald Dworkin refers to a life so conceived as that in which the person has a 'critical interest'.[10] It is this life that has ended for the demented as well as for the unconscious patient. And it is this life and only this that is of value to him. We, society as a whole, must urgently turn our attention to the needs of those whose whole system, both the physical and the mental aspects of it, has collapsed irremediably. We must ask how we are to act in their best interest, recognizing that our concept of the human organism has changed over the years, and we cannot separate their eternal soul or spirit from their corporeal existence. Better palliative care must, as a matter of course, be part of the answer, but only part. Our changed and changing view of human nature should allow us to address the question we have hitherto mostly shied away from: is continued life always in the best interest of the irredeemably suffering or demented patient? Of course if a patient, whatever he suffers, wants to stay alive, then his interests are best served by enabling him to do so as comfortably as possible. But what if he does not? Suppose he is beyond expressing any wishes or feelings at all? Or none except those of distress and misery? Faced with the spectacle of such a patient, we should not insist on the value of life, but rather on the value of that person whose life it was, but who has now lost and will never recover the sense of self that gave his life meaning. We should be more inclined than once we were to recognize that one whose body (including his brain) is fast disintegrating, though in one sense he is the same person whose name and whose history we know, in a crucial sense is not the same person. His best interests may be different from his interests when he was still leading a coherent purposeful autobiographical life. We should in time be prepared to contemplate not merely allowing him to die by withholding treatment if he falls ill, but actually and compassionately causing his death.

This, we have suggested, lies in the future. Society, though uneasy about the present law, is not ready to allow medical intervention to terminate life deliberately, except in extreme cases, such as that of Bland, or Ms B. A change in this direction is doubtless exactly what Lord Habgood so much dreads. If such acts were condoned (by, for example, a change in the law of murder) then we would be within sight of allowing euthanasia for those people whose life no longer had any meaning, even if they were not terminally ill. For the present, we must be content with palliative care for those who cannot ask to die, however poor the quality of their life, unless they have had the chance to make their wishes known through advance decisions, or their relatives or advocates bring their case to court. But we should begin to contemplate the fact that this solution may not be acceptable for ever. (That the improvement of palliative care, an agreed goal for the present, will in future, with our rapidly ageing population, become an economically unsustainable burden is perhaps something that may be left to the next generation of moralists.)

In any case, what we may or may not do now in the interests of those who are beyond requesting death, or who have not made their wishes known in advance should not be allowed to dictate what we may do in the best interests of those who rationally and soberly ask for assistance to die, either immediately, or when they are ready. We must address Baroness Richardson's question: by what moral argument can we justify insisting on keeping alive those people who sincerely want to die, when their life is, in their own eyes, not worth preserving? The thought behind the legislation in the Netherlands, in Belgium, and in the State of Oregon is that there can be no such moral justification. The more we come to accept the responsibility we already have in the matter of living and dying, the more certain it is that another Bill such as Lord Joffe's recently rejected Bill will be introduced both in the UK and elsewhere in the world. We believe that society must be ready for this.

We must therefore concentrate on and, as it were, advertise the fact that it is not irrational or morally wrong for people in some situations to be, like poor Keats, 'half in love with easeful death'. We must all, including priests, doctors, and lawyers, come to believe that deaths can be either good or bad, and that a good death is a real possibility, something that should not be denied to anyone. Where possible, the person facing his own death must decide when his death would be good, when it would be coherent with the story of his life as he lived it, as a proper and a fitting end. Ronald Dworkin suggested that most people want to express their conviction that life has had a value because of what life made it possible for them to do and feel.[11] They detest the idea that their death might express the opposite idea that mere biological life, or hanging on for the sake of it, has an independent value. The relief from physical pain may be a part of the motivation of those who beg for death in the last weeks or months of their lives; but it is probably not the whole of it. They, like those who make advance decisions, may also be motivated by the desire not to spoil the idea of the life they have lived by lingering on in a state of hopeless dependence and lack of dignity. We must accustom ourselves (as we should without difficulty be able to do) to the idea that we are mortal: that death is inevitable and sometimes to be welcomed. Even doctors must allow that, if death is the enemy, it is their patient, not they themselves who is under attack, as death approaches. It is the patient who may seek to choose his time to surrender. He need not be 'killed', if this means wrongfully killed; but he should be helped to die well.

Finally, we must address yet again what lies behind our fear of the slippery slope. Any of us who have a respect for the rule of law, not lawyers alone, understand that the law must apply universally to all who fall within its scope. If I am a motorist, I must license and insure my car. The only way to escape the force of this law, the penalties for non-compliance, is to give up my car and cease to be a motorist. If one motorist is excused, perhaps out of pity, because his car is crucial to his work, then we shall all demand to be excused. We shall all rush down the slope, and there will be an end to the law. Justice demands that all are equally liable. And so, as we have seen, a huge obstacle in the way of changing the law, as great as the objections of religion and the medical professions, is the slippery slope argument in all its forms.

The difficulty in the way of change is that, when we think of euthanasia or even of assisted suicide, we see-saw between private and public morality, between considerations of compassion for a suffering individual, on the one hand, and those of public policy, directed to the common good, on the other. Any proposal to change the law must attempt to bridge the gap between private and public, to allow compassion a place in the public domain by defining clearly the class of persons to whom the law should apply and inserting safeguards to block the descent down the slope. We must try to devise a law that will release us from the fear of its abuse, hard though this may be to draft.

But the slippery slope may not appear so very dreadful if we can come better to face our own mortality. This may entail conceding that easeful death may be the proper end for more people than we are at present inclined to believe. No future change in legislation anywhere in the world will succeed unless it arises out of an openly acknowledged change in attitude towards the prolonging of life. But, as we have argued, our attitudes have already changed, and are changing, along with our perception of what it is to be human. We also need a changed perception of doctors, armed as they now are with technological marvels that are always increasing. Indeed, they must learn to believe of themselves, as perhaps the new generation is learning, that helping someone to die without humiliation is part of their compassionate role, their age-old role as the easers of suffering and, at the end, the easers of death. In this way we may, as time goes on, introduce compassion into the laws that govern the end of life.

# Notes and References

## Introduction

1. For simplicity we have used male pronouns but in most situations this could equally well refer to a female patient or doctor.
2. For an authoritative discussion of the Dutch plea of necessity see Penney Lewis, *Assisted Dying and Legal Change* (OUP, 2007), ch. 6.
3. *Select Committee of the House of Lords on the Assisted Dying for the Terminally Ill Bill* (HL Paper no. 86, 2 vols., HMSO, Apr. 2005), i. *Report*; ii. *Evidence*.
4. Ibid. i, para 11, p. 12.

## Chapter 1

1. T. L. Beauchamp and J. C. Childress, *Principles of Biomedical Ethics* (4th edn. OUP, 1994).
2. *Pretty v. United Kingdom* (application 2346/02) [2002] 2 FLR 45.
3. Hansard, HL (10 Oct. 1995), col. 109.
4. *HL Assisted Dying*, ii, q. 913, p. 563.
5. *The Times* (13 Jan. 2007).
6. *HL Assisted Dying*, ii, q. 15756, p. 493.
7. Law Commission, *Murder, Manslaughter and Infanticide* (Law Com. No. 304, 2006), para. 7.29.

## Notes and References

### Chapter 2

1. *Rodriguez* v. *A-G of British Columbia* (1993) 107 DLR (4th) 342.
2. Dr Legemaate, *HL Assisted Dying*, ii, q. 1283, p. 416.
3. *Nancy B* v. *Hotel-Dieu de Quebec* (1992) 86 DLR (4th) 385.
4. *Ms B* v. *NHS Hospital Trust* [2002] 2 All ER 449.

### Chapter 3

1. *HL Assisted Dying*, ii, q. 1285, p. 411.
2. *Re C* (adult: refusal of medical treatment) [1994] 1 All ER 819.
3. *R* v. *SS and others* (2 Feb. 2005).
4. Katharine Graham, *Personal History* (Alfred A. Kopf, 1997).
5. *Philosophy, Psychology and Psychiatry*, 5/2 (June 1998).

### Chapter 4

1. J. A. Roberson, *Stanford Law Review*, 27 (1975), 213
2. See H. Kuhse and P. Singer, *Should the Baby Live? The Problem of Handicapped Infants* (OUP, 1985).
3. *Critical Care Decisions in Foetal and Neonatal Medicine: Ethical Issues* (Nuffield Council of Bioethics, July 2006).
4. *Lancet* (9 Aug. 1986), 328.
5. John J. Paris, Neil Graham, Michael D. Schreiber, and Michel Goodwin, *Cambridge Quarterly of Healthcare Ethics* (Spring 2006), 147sqq.
6. *An NHS Health Trust* v. *B* [2006] E44c 50.
7. Sheila Mclean, *Old Law, New Medicine* (Pandora, 1999), 121.
8. *R* v. *Arthur* (1981) 12 BMLR 1.
9. *Critical Care Decisions*, 20.

### Chapter 5

1. *Observer* (2 Mar. 2005).
2. *Airedale NHS Trust* v. *Bland* [1993] 1 All ER 821.

3. Ronald Dworkin, *Life's Dominion* (HarperCollins, 1993), 210sqq.

4. Aristotle, *Nicomachean Ethics*, book 2.

5. Hansard, HL (17 Mar. 2005), cols. 1450-2.

6. Alan Bennett, *Untold Stories* (Faber, 2005), 115sqq.

## Chapter 6

1. *HL Assisted Dying*, ii. 32.

2. Patrick Devlin, *The Enforcement of Morals* (OUP, 1965), 6.

3. *HL Assisted Dying*, ii. 488sqq.

4. Ibid. 507.

5. Jonathan Glover, *Causing Death and Saving Lives* (Penguin, 1977), 101.

6. Father Francis Marsden, 'Legalising Euthanasia Turns Carers into Killers', *Catholic Times* (2 Apr. 2006).

7. Hansard, HL (19 Apr. 2007), cols. 357-8.

## Chapter 7

1. Hansard, HL (10 Oct. 2005), col. 5.

2. James Rachels, *The End of Life: Euthanasia and Morality* (OUP, 1996).

3. Miriam Cosic, *The Right to Die: An Examination of the Euthanasia Debate* (New Holland, 2003), 164.

4. Quoted ibid. 164.

5. *HL Assisted Dying*, ii. 131.

6. See e.g. evidence to the Select Committee (ibid. 705) submitted by the Linacre Centre for Healthcare Ethics: 'In the Netherlands we see an extension of euthanasia to those who are mentally ill...and its extension to those who are unable to consent'.

7. Penney Lewis, *Assisted Dying and Legal Change* (OUP, 2007), 186.

8. Clive Seale, 'Characteristics of End of Life Decisions Made by Medical Practitioners', *Palliative Medicine* (2004), 653-9.

9. Nigel Biggar, *Aiming to Kill: The Ethics of Assisted Suicide and Euthanasia* (Darton, Longman & Todd, 2004), 169.

10. M. P. Battin, Agnes van der Heide, Linda Ganzini, Gerrit van der Wal, and Bregje D. Onwuteaka-Philipsen, 'Legal Physician-Assisted Dying in Oregon and the Netherlands: Evidence Concerning the Impact on Patients in "Vulnerable" Groups', *Journal of Medical Ethics*, 33 (2007), 591-7.

*Chapter 8*

1. James Rachels, 'Active and Passive Euthanasia', *New England Journal of Medicine*, 292 (1975), 78-80.
2. J. S. Mill, *Systems of Logic* (1843), book III, ch. 5.
3. See Ch. 2 n. 4.
4. K. Dunphy, 'Futilitarianism: Knowing How Much is Enough in End-of-Life Health Care', *New England Journal of Medicine*, 337/17 (23 Oct. 1997), 1236-9.
5. Fiona Randall and R. S. Downie, *The Philosophy of Palliative Care: Critique and Reconstruction* (OUP, 2006).

*Chapter 9*

1. M. Richards, Keynote Address on National Initiative in End of Life Care: Conference; 'Current Issues in Palliative Care', Institute of Physics, London, 2 May 2007.
2. S. Murray, A. Sheikh, and K. Thomas, 'Advance Care Planning in Primary Care', editorial, *BMJ* 333 (2006), 868-9.
3. Anne-Mei The, Tony Hak, Gerard Koeter, and Gerrit van der Wal, 'Collusion in Doctor–Patient Communication about Imminent Death: An Ethnographic Study', *BMJ* 321 (2000), 1376-81.
4. J. A. Rietjens, A. van der Heide, B. D. Onwuteaka-Phillipsen, P. J. Vander Maas, and G. Van de Wal, 'A Comparison of Attitudes towards End-of-Life Decisions: Survey among the Dutch General Public and Physicians', *Social Science and Medicine*, 61/8 (2005), 1723-32.

5. D. Eddy, 'A Conversation with my Mother', *Journal of the American Medical Association*, 272/3 (1994), 179–81. L. A. Printz, 'Terminal Dehydration: A Compassionate Treatment', *Archives of Internal Medicine*, 152 (1992), 697–700. T. E. Quill, B. Coombs Lee, and S. Nunn, 'Palliative Treatments of Last Resort: Choosing the Least Harmful Alternative', *Annals of Internal Medicine*, 132/6 (2000), 488–93.

6. L. A. Printz, 'Is Withholding Hydration a Valid Comfort Measure in the Terminally Ill?', *Geriatrics*, 43/11 (Nov. 1988), 84–8. J. Zerwekh, 'The Dehydration Question', *Nursing*, 83 (Jan. 1983), 47–51.

7. *Airedale NHS Trust v. Bland*, House of Lords, Judgment 4 Feb. 1993.

8. T. E. Quill, B. Lo, and D. W. Brock, 'Palliative Options of Last Resort: A Comparison of Voluntarily Stopping Eating and Drinking, Terminal Sedation, Physician-Assisted Suicide and Voluntary Active Euthanasia', *Journal of the American Medical Association*, 278 (1997), 2099–2104.

9. H. C. Muller-Busch, I. Andres, and T. Jehser, 'Sedation in Palliative Care: A Critical Analysis of 7 Years' Experience', *BMC (BioMed Central) Palliat Care*, 2/2 (2003). Published online 13 May 2003.

10. K. G. Wilson et al, 'Suffering with Advanced Cancer', *Journal of Clinical Oncology*, 25/13 (2007) 1691–97.

11. R. L. Fainsiger, A. Waller, M. Bercovici, K. Bengston, W. Landman, M. Hosking, J. M. Nunez-Alarte, and D. deMoissac, 'A Multicentre International Study of Sedation in Terminally Ill Patients', *Palliative Medicine*, 14 (2000), 257–65.

12. J. Porta Sales, Y. Catala Bore, and G. Estibalez, 'A Multi-Centred Trial in Sedation of the Terminally Ill', *Medicina Paliativa*, 6/4 (1999), 153–8 (Spanish).

13. N. Sykes and A. Thorn, 'The Use of Opioids and Sedatives at the End of Life', *Lancet Oncology*, 4 (2003), 312–18.

14. N. Sykes and A. Thorn, 'Sedative Use in the Last Week of Life and the Implications for End-of-Life Decision Making', *Archives of Internal Medicine*, 163 (2003), 341–4.

## Notes and References

15. N. Sykes, 'Morphine Kills the Pain Not the Patient', *The Lancet on Line*, 369 (27 Apr. 2007), 1325-6 (www.thelancet.com).

16. Dr Richard Leman giving evidence concerning the Death with Dignity programme in Oregon USA: *HL Assisted Dying*, ii. *Evidence* (9 Dec. 2004), 260.

17. H. Hendin, 'Seduced by Death: Doctors, Patients and the Dutch Cure', *Issues in Law and Medicine*, 10/2 (1994), 123-68.

18. A. van der Heide, B. D. Onwuteaka-Philipsen, M. L. Rurup, H. M. Buiting, J. J. van Delden, J. E. Hanssen-deWolf, A. G. Janssen, H. R. Pasman, J. A. Rietjens, C. J. Prins, I. M. Deerenberg, J. K. Gevers, P. J. van der Maas, and G. van der Wal, 'End of Life Practices in the Netherlands under the Euthanasia Act', *New England Journal of Medicine*, 356/19 (May 2007), 1957-65 (www.NEJM.org).

19. I. Haverkate, A. van der Heide, B. D. Onwuteaka-Phillipsen, P. J. van der Maas, and G. van de Wal, 'The Emotional Impact on Physicians of Hastening the Death of a Patient', *Medical Journal of Australia*, 175 (2001), 519 22.

20. Baroness Thomas of Walliswood, quoting conversations with doctors in Holland: *HL Assisted Dying*, ii (9 Dec.2004), 538.

21. K. L. Obstein, G. Kimsma, and T. Chambers, 'Practicing Euthanasia: The Perspective of Physicians', *Journal of Medical Ethics*, 15/2 (2004), 223-31.

22. E. J. Emannuel, E. Daniels, D. Fairclough, and B. R. Clarridge, 'The Practice of Euthanasia and Physician-Assisted Suicide in the United States: Adherence to Proposed Safeguards and Effects on Physicians', *Journal of the American Medical Association*, 280/6 (1998), 507-13.

23. T. E. Quill, 'Opening the Black Box: Physicians' Inner Responses to Patients' Requests for Physician-Assisted Death', editorial, *Journal of Palliative Medicine*, 7/3 (2004), 469-71.

24. D. Meier, C.-A. Emmons, S. Wallenstein, T. Quill, R. S. Morrison, and C. K. Cassel, 'A National Survey of Physician-Assisted Suicide

and Euthanasia in the United States', *New England Journal of Medicine*, 338/17 (1998), 1193-1201.

25. K. L. Vaux, 'Debbie's Dying: Mercy Killing and the Good Death', letter, *Journal of the American Medical Association*, 259/14 (1988), 2140-1.
26. C. Clark and G. Kimsma, '"Medical Friendships" in Assisted Dying', *Cambridge Quarterly of Healthcare Ethics*, 13 (2004), 61-7.
27. Dr John Bos (surgical oncologist practising in Holland): *HL Assisted Dying*, ii (16 Dec. 2004), p. 423.

*Chapter 10*

1. Hansard, HL (10 Oct. 2005), cols. 134-5.
2. *Observer* (12 Feb. 2006).
3. P. F. Strawson, *Individuals: An Essay in Descriptive Metaphysics* (Methuen, 1959), ch. 3.
4. J.-P. Sartre, 'Une idée fondamentale de la phenomenologie de Husserl: L'Intentionalité', *Situations*, 1 (Gallimard, 1947).
5. Gilbert Ryle, *The Concept of Mind* (Hutchinson, 1949), *passim.*
6. Ludwig Wittgenstein, *Philosophical Investigations*, tr. G. E. M. Anscombe (Blackwell, 1959), paras 275-397.
7. *HL Assisted Dying*, ii. 66sqq.
8. Hansard, HL (12 May 2006), cols. 1244-5.
9. British Medical Association, *Withholding and Withdrawing Life-Prolonging Medical Treatment: Guidance for Decision-Making* (BMJ Books, rev. edn. 2001).
10. Ronald Dworkin, *Life's Dominion* (HarperCollins, 1992), 215.
11. Ibid. 212.

# Index

# Index

# Index

# Index